Retirement Activity Book

Activity Book

For The Newly Retired

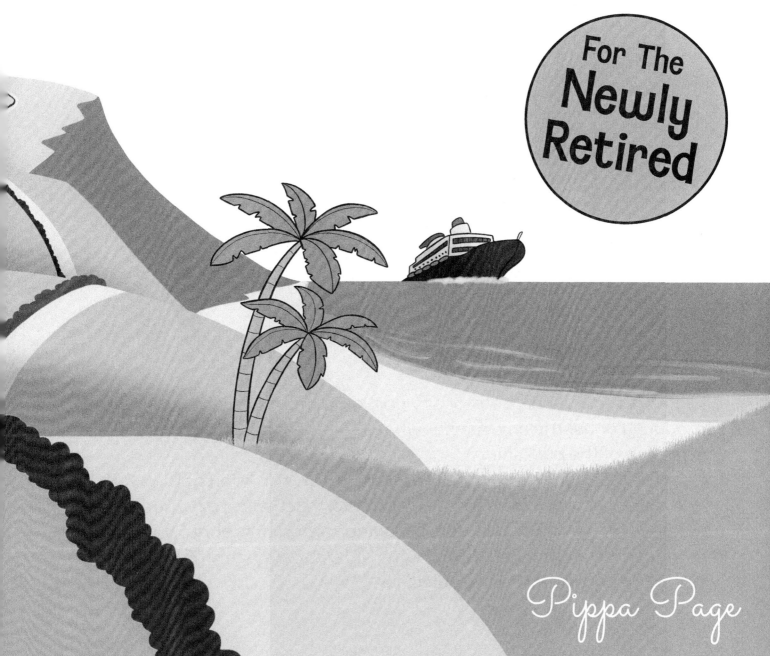

Pippa Page

Contents

Puzzle Type	Page Number
Billiard Balls	29,87,100,
Calculations	22,44,66,82,102,
Crossword	42,52,68,80,98,108,124
Cryptogram	7,38,64,65,79,88,103,
Cryptogram Grid	20,50,96,120,
Guess The Country	25,73,
Guess The Flag	30,
Maze	18,37,74,90,116,
Number Squares	41,72,130,
Pairs	17,39,56,104,129,
Rebus	40,
Roman Numerals	16,45,55,61,75,106,
Safe Code	31,70,110,
Sudoku	10,19,32,76,94,118,
Trivia Quiz	14,34,62,92,112,
What Goes Where	8,13,27,46,84,114,119,123,
Word Association	9,48,60,86,89,107,122,132,
Word Builder	24,54,78,95,126,
Word Scramble	28,58,77,111,131,
Word Search	6,12,26,36,49,57,67,83,91,105, 117,128,
Answers & Solutions	134

"Retirement is a blank sheet of paper. It is a chance to redesign your life into something new and different."

Patrick Foley

"There is a whole new kind of life ahead, full of experiences just waiting to happen. Some call it retirement. I call it bliss."

Betty Sullivan

Congratulations on your well-deserved retirement!

It's time to embark on a new adventure filled with relaxation, fun, and mental stimulation. Celebrate your newfound freedom and embrace your golden years with this perfect companion for your retirement journey, offering a delightful mix of fun trivia, brain-teasing challenges and a sprinkling of inspirational quotes and funny retirement quips to keep you smiling.

In the pages that follow you will find over 120 diverse puzzles including engaging word searches, challenging crosswords, intriguing sudoku puzzles, fascinating trivia quizzes, mind-bending mazes, clever word scrambles, stimulating maths problems and more.

Whether you're looking to establish a new daily routine, pass the time on a relaxing afternoon, or challenge yourself to learn something new, this book has something for everyone. With varying difficulty levels, you can progress at your own pace and celebrate your achievements along the way. You can find all the answers and solutions at the back of the book.

Happy Retirement!

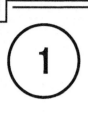

70s & 80s Action Movies

Remember these action flicks?
Find each movie title in the grid!

```
R R A I D E R S O F T H E L O S T A R K
L C A F I R S T B L O O D L R Z A B O R
F I S T O F F U R Y B K M O N S A K B T
H S O F N X P O Q U H L T E U S C N O H
S F Z O E D Y B R Y E A I N F E O N C E
A B N D H M T B R C D L O I A N M Q O T
S T A R W A R S R E A I I C A W M J P E
O D F L J D A O R O S U P E R M A N K R
N I I T U M F P B A W C W G S L N I L M
B E N R B A L I V E A N D L E T D I E I
F H M C T X K N J N T J N E O O O W O N
I A T L N Y I S U D D E N I M P A C T A
L R E L E T H A L W E A P O N G N W E T
D D N H S B B A T M A N E X L U X R B O
P O Z Q M O O N R A K E R X L N U B V R
H B Z O F E N T E R T H E D R A G O N F
O N M X A P O C A L Y P S E N O W W Y F
```

FIST OF FURY   ROBOCOP   ALIEN   DIE HARD   TRUE LIES   TOP GUN

MOONRAKER   MAD MAX   FIRST BLOOD   SUDDEN IMPACT   ENTER THE DRAGON

DIRTY HARRY   THE TERMINATOR   RAIDERS OF THE LOST ARK   COMMANDO

STAR WARS   APOCALYPSE NOW   SUPERMAN   DELTA FORCE   LETHAL WEAPON

LIVE AND LET DIE   BATMAN   PREDATOR   FOXY BROWN   INVASION USA

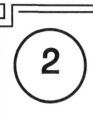

Cryptogram

2

Decrypt the names of these popular global newspapers using the key below.

A	B	C	D	E	F	G	H	I	J	K	L	M
21	23	4	17	5	20	12	8	26	6	9	15	1

N	O	P	Q	R	S	T	U	V	W	X	Y	Z
7	25	24	16	10	19	18	13	3	11	22	14	2

Ⓐ

18	8	5

11	21	19	8	26	7	12	18	25	7

24	25	19	18

Ⓑ

18	8	5

12	13	21	10	17	26	21	7

Ⓒ

18	8	5

18	25	10	25	7	18	25

19	18	21	10

What Goes Where?

3

Group the words below into the 3 categories given.

Where did these beverages originate?

Tequila   Perrier   Cognac

Spritz   Espresso   Cappuccino

Margarita   Champagne

FRANCE

ITALY

MEXICO

Word Association

4

Guess the thing, event, or person associated with the group of 3 words

(A)
AUTUMN
WISHBONE
FAMILY

....

(B)
NEW YORK
HENDRIX
FLOWER POWER

....

(C)
COFFEE
COCA-COLA
RED BULL

....

(D)
ROWLAND H. MACY
SAM WALTON
CHARLES H. HARROD

....

(E)
BOB KANE
JACK KIRBY
JERRY SIEGEL

....

5

Fill each square with a number from 1 to 9 without repeating a number in the vertical or horizontal columns.

Sudoku 1

5			8			2	9	
				2				
4			7	5		3		
	9	2			3	4		
				9			6	
				8				
						9		2
		3					4	
	6					7	8	

Sudoku 2

					5		7	
	9							
				6		1		5
						8		
2	5		8					4
7			5				6	2
	6	7		9	2			
				2				8
4	2	5						

Sudoku 3

	5						4	
	9		4					
	8							6
3						8		5
			5					
				2	6			9
8			7					2
6	2		5	9		4		
9				8			7	

Sudoku 4

3					8			
1		5		4	2			
8	6		7					
4			3					
5		2					8	6
6			8		7	2	1	
	8		2	3	5	6	4	
							7	

"When a man retires, his wife gets twice as much husband for half as much money."

Chi Chi Rodriguez

Popular Magazines

Find each of these popular magazines in the grid below.

```
P O P U L A R M E C H A N I C S H G H F
N E W N K D C O S M O P O L I T A N P A
N G O O D H O U S E K E E P I N G W X M
L U X W T V O G U E F R O N T I E R S I
G T R A D I O T I M E S A X E X A V E L
W N O F C L M N B B C G O O D F O O D Y
E E L I C K Q E Y C E H B M G Z Q L X C
E R L F H O M E S A N D G A R D E N S I
C E I A M E N S H E A L T H P I S F Y R
D A N A T I O N A L G E O G R A P H I C
A D G N U G L C Q Z L N E W S W E E K L
A E S F B E P O P U L A R S C I E N C E
X R T H E E C O N O M I S T X R U H P U
S P O R T S I L L U S T R A T E D U U Y
V A N I T Y F A I R N L D Q Y D U E V E
M P E O P L E W F O R B E S M P L I X W
Z V S E V E N T E E N H O Q G V A I F G
```

MEN'S HEALTH   PEOPLE   NATIONAL GEOGRAPHIC   VANITY FAIR   NEWSWEEK

SEVENTEEN   UTNE READER   POPULAR MECHANICS   POPULAR SCIENCE

WIRED   LIFE   COSMOPOLITAN   GOOD HOUSEKEEPING   VOGUE   FAMILY CIRCLE

RADIO TIMES   SPORTS ILLUSTRATED   HOMES AND GARDENS   THE ECONOMIST

ROLLING STONE   FORBES   TIME   BBC GOOD FOOD   FRONTIERS   DELICIOUS

What Goes Where?

7

Group the words below into the 3 categories given.

Match the jargon to the hobby.

Banding Wheel   **Bar clamp**   **Bevel**

Magic ring   **Ceramic glaze**

Slip stitch   **Front post**   **Kiln**

CROCHET   WOODWORKING   POTTERY

Trivia

Test your knowledge of the decades you've lived through!

1. In what year did humans first set foot on the moon?
a) 1963
b) 1965
c) 1969
d) 1971

2. Which TV show featured Archie Bunker?
a) M*A*S*H
b) All in the Family
c) The Waltons
d) Happy Days

3. Who played James Bond in "Goldfinger" (1964)?
a) Pierce Brosnan
b) Roger Moore
c) Timothy Dalton
d) Sean Connery

4. What sport did Martina Navratilova play?
a) Soccer
b) Baseball
c) Basketball
d) Tennis

5. In what year did the Berlin Wall fall?
a) 1985
b) 1991
c) 1989
d) 1993

6. What was the first home video game console?
a) Magnavox Odyssey
b) Atari 2600
c) Nintendo NES
d) Sega Genesis

7. Which Beatle released a solo album called "All Things Must Pass"?
a) John Lennon
b) Paul McCartney
c) George Harrison
d) Ringo Starr

8. Who became the Prime Minister of the UK in 1979?
a) Harold Wilson
b) Margaret Thatcher
c) Edward Heath
d) James Callaghan

9. Which car was known as the "People's Car"?
a) Volkswagen Beetle
b) Ford Mustang
c) Chevrolet Camaro
d) Mini Cooper

10. Who wrote "One Hundred Years of Solitude"?
a) J.R.R. Tolkien
b) Gabriel García Márquez
c) George Orwell
d) Agatha Christie

Roman Numerals Calculations

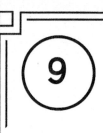

9

How well do you know the Roman numerals?
Calculate the value of each set of numerals
below.

A   XXIV + XVI   =

B   L – XXIII   =

C   XII × III   =

D   XC ÷ V   =

E   (L + XX) – (X × II)   =

F   C – LX + XXXIV   =

Skeletal Smarts

10

Match the bones to their medical names.

SHOULDER BLADE	TIBIA
KNEECAP	PELVIS
FINGER BONES	COCCYX
COLLAR BONE	SCAPULA
HIPS	STERNUM
SHIN	ORBIT
TAILBONE	PHALANGES
BREASTBONE	MANDIBLE
JAW BONE	CLAVICLE
EYE SOCKET	PATELLA

Maze

11

Find your way through this maze!

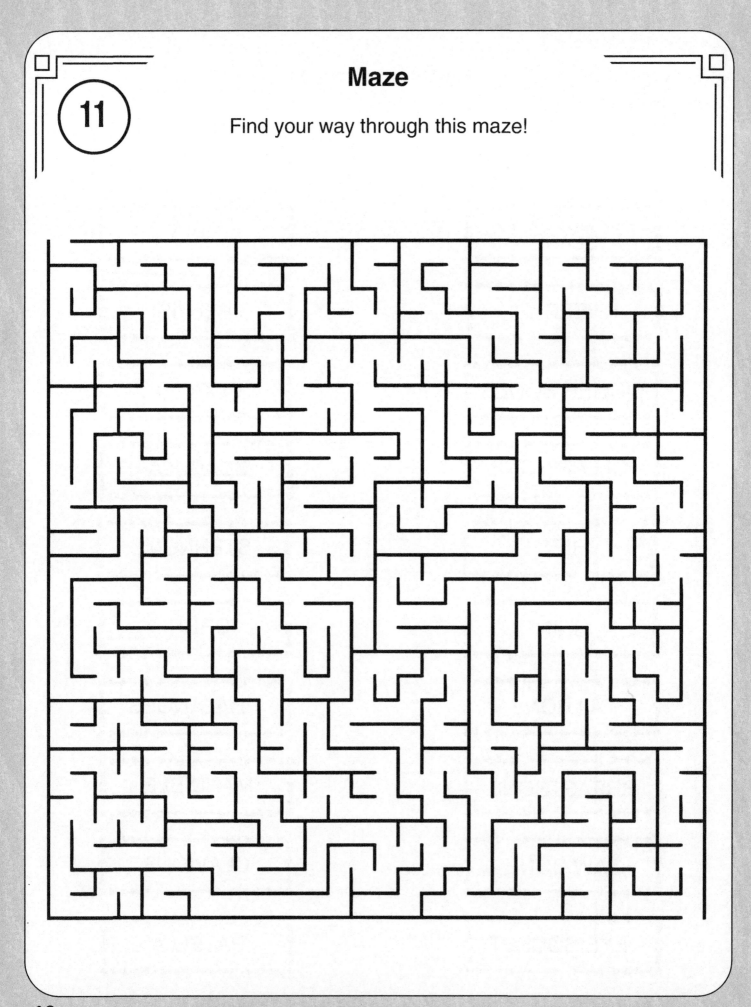

Sudoku

12

Fill each square with a number from 1 to 9 without repeating a number in the vertical or horizontal columns.

Sudoku 5

			3				1	9
				5				
			2	5		3		
9		1	4			8		
							7	
8			7			3		
	2	9				8		
			1	4				
		3				7		5

Sudoku 6

6	1		2					
						1	8	
			5	7		3		6
			5		2			
			9			2	3	8
9								
7							2	
						1		6
			1				7	9

Sudoku 7

	3		2		8			9
			3			4		
6	9	1						
	7		3	2				
8			4		9	3		
			8		6			4
9	1							
		7						
3	8	2						6

Sudoku 8

5			2					
6	1	4	9	8				2
			4					8
	9	1			7	8		4
			6		4			9
2								
			9	1				5
			7			4		
						1		

Cryptogram

Using the clues, solve the puzzle to reveal an activity a retiree might love.

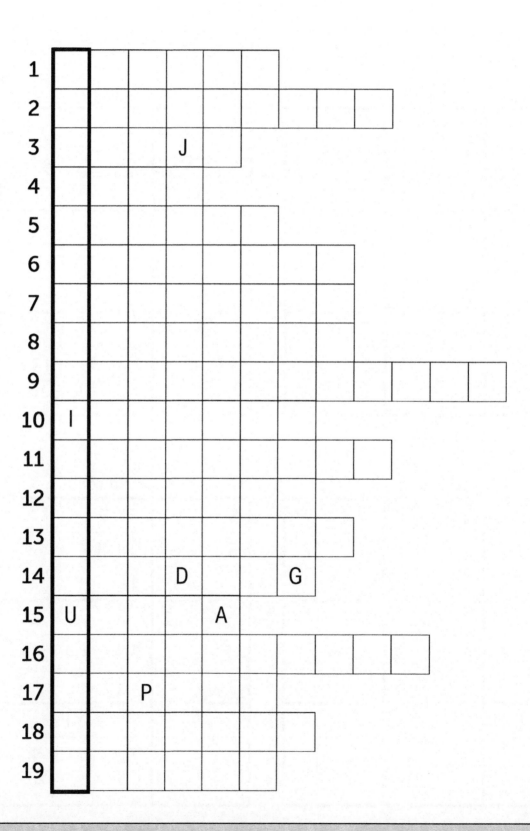

Guess the cities and country capitals.

1. Capital city of Portugal

2. Scotland's capital.

3. Capital city of Nigeria.

4. Vatican City is in this city.

5. Capital of the Bahamas.

6. Capital of the UAE.

7. India's capital city.

8. Capital city of Alberta, Canada.

9. Home of the White House and U.S Capitol?

10. Famous Brazilian city.

11. U.S state bordered by New York and Pennsylvania.

12. Costa Rica's capital.

13. France's "Pink City".

14. Town on the River Thames.

15. Town in New York State.

16. Capital city of Mexico.

17. City and county in Texas.

18. Capital city of Kenya.

19. Taiwan's capital.

Calculation Questions

14

Solve the math problems below.

1. Matthew's pension pays $2,500 per month, how much would he have gotten from January 2017 to January 2023?

2. Jessica invests $10,000 in a retirement fund that grows at an average annual rate of 6%, how much will she have after 20 years?

3. Alex purchases an annuity that pays $800 per month for 20 years, how much will he receive in total over the annuity's lifetime?

4. Joan's employer matches 50% of her 401(k) contributions up to 6% of her salary. She earns $60,000 annually. How much should she contribute annually to get the 6% match?

5. Luke's spends $500 a month on healthcare. His healthcare expenses are expected to increase by 3% each year due to inflation. How much will his monthly healthcare expenses be after 5 years?

"Retirement is not in my vocabulary. They aren't going to get rid of me that way."

Betty White

Word Builder

Can you put these letter groups together to form 9-letter words associated with outer space?

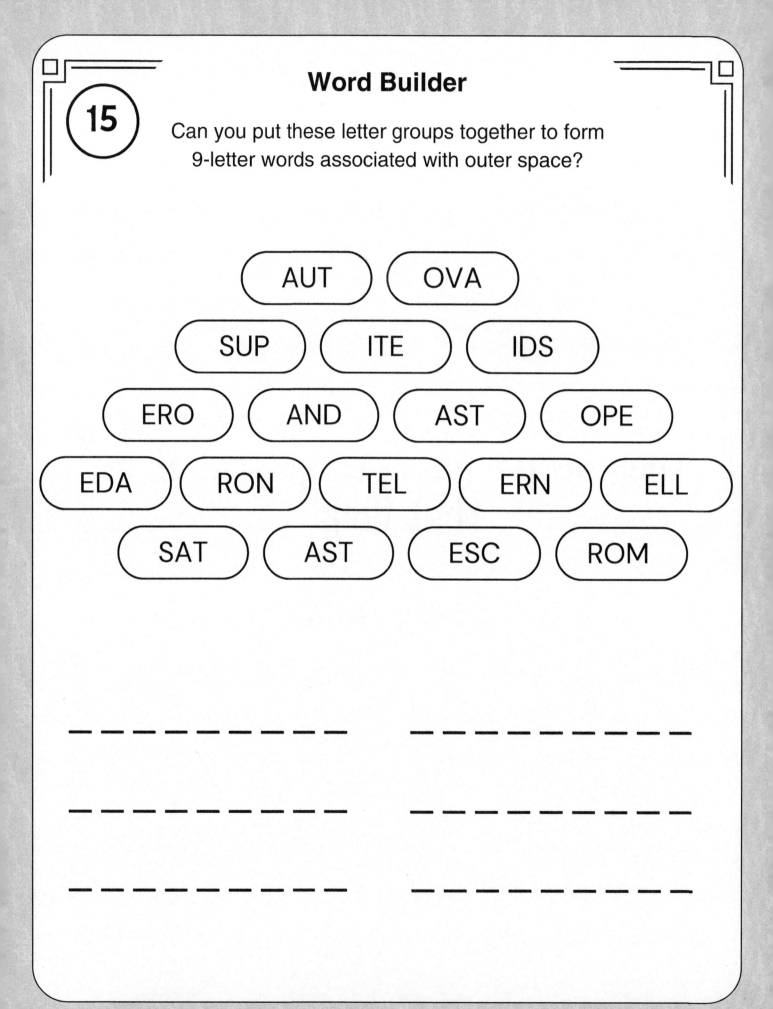

AUT   OVA

SUP   ITE   IDS

ERO   AND   AST   OPE

EDA   RON   TEL   ERN   ELL

SAT   AST   ESC   ROM

_____   _____

_____   _____

_____   _____

Guess the Country

Test your geography knowledge - identify the countries below!

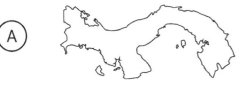

(A) LOCATION: Central America

....

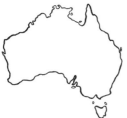

(B) LOCATION: Oceania

....

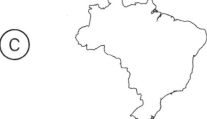

(C) LOCATION: South America

....

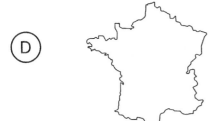

(D) LOCATION: Western Europe

....

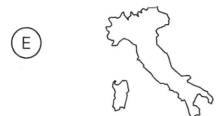

(E) LOCATION: South-central Europe

....

Gardening

17

Find the words associated with gardening in the grid below.

```
I  D  P  Z  F  R  U  I  T  I  F  X  G  H  L  N  A  R  A  I
H  Y  T  P  L  X  S  U  N  L  I  G  H  T  G  M  U  E  G  X
F  G  Z  M  O  Z  G  E  P  S  B  P  X  E  R  K  H  K  Q  I
F  D  B  J  W  L  O  T  E  V  E  R  G  R  E  E  N  U  H  R
O  A  A  C  E  W  L  D  R  D  A  V  E  G  E  T  A  B  L  E
E  S  X  R  R  H  U  I  E  B  L  F  D  K  N  H  B  T  L  K
T  H  O  W  S  E  Y  Z  N  N  C  I  O  H  H  R  D  W  J  M
L  E  R  I  D  E  V  G  N  A  H  L  N  F  O  R  K  F  R  Z
M  A  X  A  L  L  U  T  I  P  T  A  M  G  U  T  P  P  P  D
V  R  P  W  A  B  H  R  A  Q  D  I  I  W  S  A  L  S  O  N
Y  S  N  W  Y  A  J  O  L  B  A  I  O  O  E  I  P  N  O  W
V  M  B  D  L  R  Y  W  S  W  R  V  P  N  L  E  K  X  N  L
L  V  A  D  G  R  F  E  D  E  O  M  L  G  C  W  D  S  T  M
P  L  N  N  Z  O  M  L  G  H  O  P  R  U  N  E  R  S  Z  P
G  A  E  O  U  W  R  K  E  C  T  P  H  E  P  K  B  K  O  Y
T  W  A  T  E  R  I  N  G  C  A  N  D  E  E  H  L  Z  C  H
Z  I  I  W  Y  S  E  E  D  S  D  Q  O  W  F  U  Y  R  O  T
```

FLOWERS   GREENHOUSE   FORK   PRUNERS   EVERGREEN

APHID   SHEARS   LADYBUG   SEEDLINGS   WEEDS   SPADE   TROWEL   MANURE

WATERING CAN   ROOT   SEEDS   SUNLIGHT   FRUIT   POLLINATION   HOSE

PERENNIALS   VEGETABLE   COMPOST   WHEELBARROW   SOIL

What Goes Where?

18

Group the words below into the 3
categories given.

Sort these movies into the correct genre.

The Birds   The Wiz   Notting Hill

Mystic Pizza   The Omen

Moonstruck   Time Bandits   Suspiria

HORROR

ROMANCE

FANTASY

Unscramble the Words

(19)

Unscramble the names of these cities in the Americas!

BEAUSENIORS   _ _ _ _ _ _ _ _ _ _

GLEASNOLES   _ _ _ _ _ _ _ _ _ _

ROADIEOIJNER   _ _ _ _ _ _ _ _ _ _ _ _

AAHNAV   _ _ _ _ _ _

ELANWONESR   _ _ _ _ _ _ _ _ _ _

NOVAURVEC   _ _ _ _ _ _ _ _ _

RANARAQUILLB   _ _ _ _ _ _ _

ALONTERM   _ _ _ _ _ _ _ _ _

Billiard Balls

20

Fill in the boxes to complete the calculations below.

A) 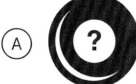 X 9 − 81 = 234

B) 45 32 / 7 = 11

C) 56 / ? + 23 = 30

D) ? + 30 X 2 = 110

E) 72 ? 18 X 3 = 18

Guess the Flag

21

Guess the country each national flag belongs to.

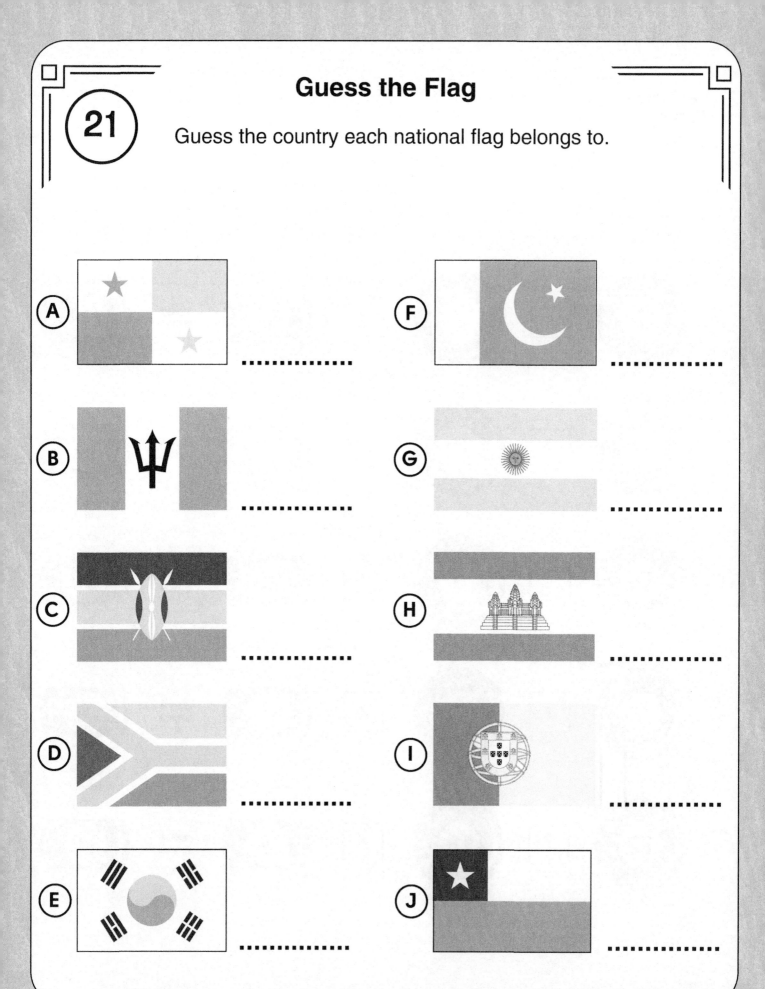

A ....

B ....

C ....

D ....

E ....

F ....

G ....

H ....

I ....

J ....

Safe Code

22

Identify the number pattern and replace the blank spaces with the correct digits to unlock the safe.

A
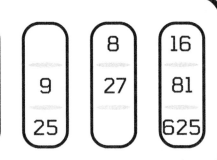

2		8	16
	9	27	81
5	25		625

B
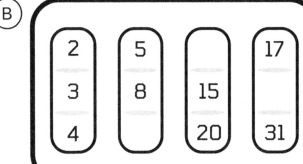

2	5		17
3	8	15	
4		20	31

C
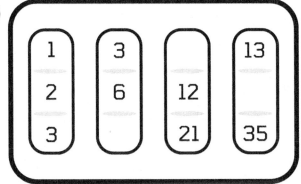

1	3		13
2	6	12	
3		21	35

D
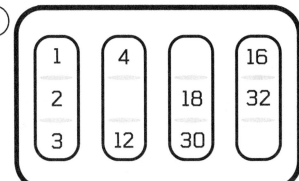

1	4		16
2		18	32
3	12	30	

Sudoku

Fill each square with a number from 1 to 9 without repeating a number in the vertical or horizontal columns.

Sudoku 9

2			1				8	6
	8	1	3					4
	4		7	6				
7			6				3	1
		6	1					
3					8			
9			8					
1	2	3	9		7			
	7			2				

Sudoku 10

			2		4			9
			9	8				4
	3	1			9	5		6
			5				4	3
			8	5		9		2
9	8		6					5
				2				
			5	3	8			

Sudoku 11

	7		8					
4		8						3
3					9		2	
			6					
8	1							
7	3			9				6
9						3		4
			9					
6		1		4	3		8	7

Sudoku 12

	4	6			9			
2		9		6			7	
			1	3				2
	7			2		9	4	
		8		4	6	7		
6								
8					3			
						1	3	
	3			9		2		

"Retirement is like a long vacation in Las Vegas. The goal is to enjoy it to the fullest, but not so fully that you run out of money."

Jonathan Clements

Trivia

Test your knowledge of the sitcoms of the 70s and 80s.

1. Who is the main character in "Happy Days"?
a) Fonzie
b) Richie Cunningham
c) Mr. C
d) Potsie Weber

2. Mike and Carol are the parents in which family?
a) Potter
b) Nelson
c) Brady
d) Smith

3. Who played "George" on "The Jeffersons"?
a) Redd Foxx
b) James Avery
c) Bill Cosby
d) Sherman Hemsley

4. What was the name of the bar in "Cheers"?
a) The White Horse
b) The Drunken Duck
c) Cheers
d) The Cozy Corner

5. Who was the neighbor on "Three's Company"?
a) Mr. Roper
b) Mr. Johnson
c) Mr. Green
d) Mr. Wilson

6. Who played Mork in "Mork & Mindy"?
a) Paul Fusco
b) Jaleel White
c) Robin Williams
d) Gary Coleman

7. Which show starred Ron Howard as Opie?
a) Happy Days
b) Leave It to Beaver
c) The Andy Griffith Show
d) The Wonder Years

8. Who played Arnold in "Diff'rent Strokes"?
a) Gary Coleman
b) Dustin Diamond
c) Emmanuel Lewis
d) Todd Bridges

9. What was the name of the oldest Brady girl?
a) Carol
b) Cindy
c) Jan
d) Marcia

10. Who played the role of Edith Bunker on "All in the Family"?
a) Betty White
b) Jean Stapleton
c) Lucille Ball
d) Carroll O'Connor

Outdoor Activities

25

Find the fun outdoor activities in the grid below.

```
U M P O K P Y O U B A R B E C U E L M X
G M Z F A K P B A C K P A C K I N G F C
H G A F T D B Q D G A R D E N I N G Z V
M O P R P F O T F C S L E D D I N G S O
A X W O K N P F P U O W A L K I N G G H
P G M A R R H I O N T T L A J B N N R Z
V P Z D Z X O S I O R H Y L H I I E O N
M N G I J J T H E I T A O Q P R M P C V
O S F N F O O I B X K B G M E D Y A K S
U A T G T T G N T L Y N A E X W N I C S
F X S N D N R G A K I C T L A A N L A
E K U D I P A K I V V N W E L T H T I I
X T R T T V P K I N E T O Q H C L I M L
T S F T V K H D G I G O L F V H L N B I
O A I H L R Y V R M B C Y C L I N G I N
R S N N O K F O P X X P M H U N T I N G
O F G E S S U E S W I M M I N G Y M G T
```

CYCLING   KAYAKING   PHOTOGRAPHY   ROCK CLIMBING

WALKING   BIRD WATCHING   SWIMMING   HUNTING   JOGGING

ORIENTEERING   YOGA   SKY DIVING   FOOTBALL   GOLF   CAMPING

FISHING   BARBECUE   RAFTING   SLEDDING   GARDENING   PAINTING

SURFING   OFF-ROADING   BACKPACKING   SAILING

Maze

26

Find your way through this maze!

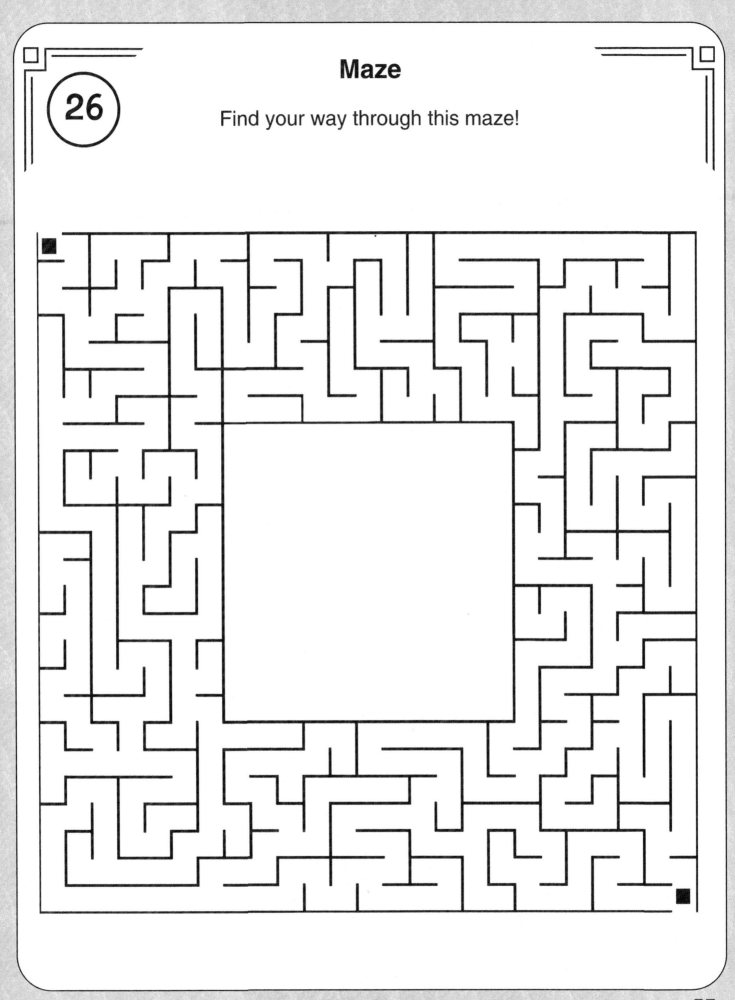

Cryptogram

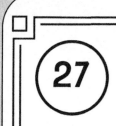

27

Decrypt the American football terms using the key below.

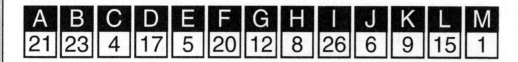

A	B	C	D	E	F	G	H	I	J	K	L	M
21	23	4	17	5	20	12	8	26	6	9	15	1

N	O	P	Q	R	S	T	U	V	W	X	Y	Z
7	25	24	16	10	19	18	13	3	11	22	14	2

(A)

26	7	18	5	10	4	5	24	18	26	25	7

(B)

10	5	17

2	25	7	5

(C)

20	21	26	10

4	21	18	4	8

World Leaders

Match these famous world leaders to their countries.

SULEIMAN	ROME
HATSHEPSUT	CANADA
AUGUSTUS	INDIA
HAMMURABI	ENGLAND
KIM CAMPBELL	OTTOMAN EMPIRE
JUAN PERÓN	BABYLON
VICTORIA	EGYPT
KWAME NKRUMAH	GHANA
INDIRA GANDHI	SPAIN
PHILIP II	ARGENTINA

Rebus Puzzle

Use the picture clues to guess the historic event that happened in the 20th century.

Ⓐ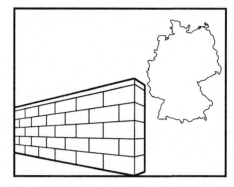

....

Ⓑ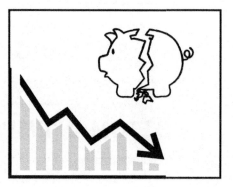

....

Ⓒ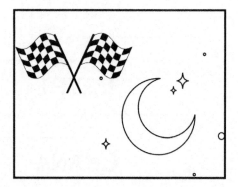

....

Ⓓ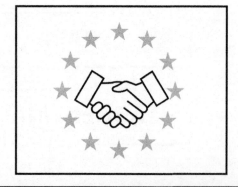

....

Number Squares

Fill in the boxes to complete the calculations below.

A (48) [+] (12) [X] (3) [?] (20) = (64)

B (84) [/] (?) [X] (5) [+] (12) = (72)

C (?) [-] (24) [/] (4) [X] (3) = (78)

D (72) [+] (16) [/] (4) [X] (?) = (84)

E (55) [/] (5) [X] (?) [+] (10) = (54)

Crossword

Use the clues to help you fill in the squares.
The theme is "At the Bakery".

Across

1. Dunkin and Krispy Kreme?

7. Gourmet cupcakes are sold here.

8. 13 buns, for example.

10. Baked good eaten with gravy in the U.S.

16. Italian ricotta-filled pastry.

18. Dole baking contest winner?

19. Dough flattener or impromptu weapon.

22. Eclair coating.

23. Flour, salt, chocolate powder, for example.

24. Custard dessert with caramelized top.

Down

2. Fermented bread starter.

3. Baking instruction?

4. Pastry dough for pies.

5. Long French bread?

6. Italian dessert with coffee and mascarpone.

9. Butter substitute?

11. Aussies' national dessert.

12. Mars Inc. or Haribo, for example.

13. French bakery specializing in bread.

14. Leavening agent used in pastries.

15. Texture and thickness of a batter.

16. Popular French pastry.

17. Process that makes dough rise.

20. Dominique Ansel or Duff Goldman?

21. Colorful French cookie.

Calculation Questions

Solve the math problems below.

1. If Greg invests $15,000 in a retirement account with an annual return rate of 5%, how much will the investment be worth after 10 years?

_ _ _ _ _ _ _

2. Carlos receives a monthly pension of $3,200. How much would he have received in total after 15 years?

_ _ _ _ _ _ _

3. Lucy plans to take a vacation every year for the next 10 years, budgeting $3,500 for each vacation. How much total will she spend on vacations over the 10 years?

_ _ _ _ _ _ _

4. Janet spends $150 per month on gardening supplies for her hobby. How much will she spend in 5 years?

_ _ _ _ _ _ _

5. If Paula receives an annual benefit of $12,000 from her investments, how much will she have received after 25 years?

_ _ _ _ _ _ _

Roman Numerals Calculations

(33)

How well do you know the Roman numerals?
Calculate the value of each set of numerals
below.

(A) XLII + XXXVII   =

(B) LXXXV – XXX   =

(C) VI × IX   =

(D) XC ÷ III   =

(E) (LIV + XX) ÷ II   =

(F) XXVII + XVIII   =

What Goes Where?

Group the words below into the 3 categories given.

Match these mountains to their continent.

Mount Stanley   **Mont Blanc**   **Matterhorn**

Kilimanjaro   **Mount Logan**

Ben Nevis   **Mount Whitney**   **Denali**

NORTH AMERICA

EUROPE

AFRICA

"Retirement is wonderful. It's doing nothing without worrying about getting caught at it."

Gene Perret

Word Association

Guess the thing, event, or person associated
with the group of 3 words

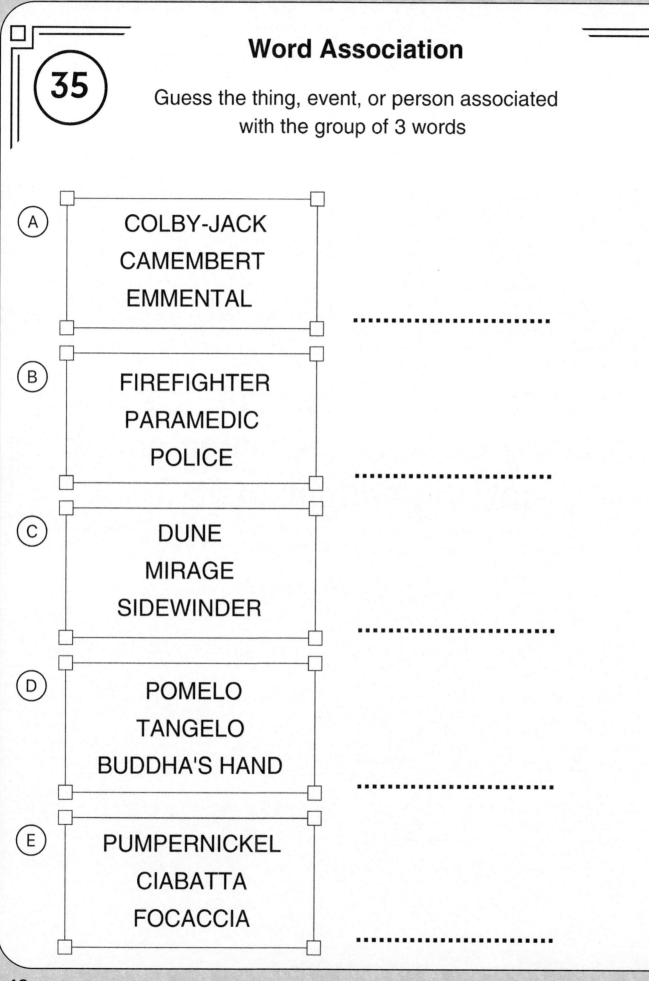

35

A
COLBY-JACK
CAMEMBERT
EMMENTAL

....

B
FIREFIGHTER
PARAMEDIC
POLICE

....

C
DUNE
MIRAGE
SIDEWINDER

....

D
POMELO
TANGELO
BUDDHA'S HAND

....

E
PUMPERNICKEL
CIABATTA
FOCACCIA

....

Art

Get creative and find these art-related
words in the grid below.

```
H G D Q P A L E T T E K N I F E B W F N
C L A Y F P W W C Y S U R R E A L I S M
Z U P O R T R A I T L X E F I R E K S E
B N B I Y Q R E N A I S S A N C E M R I
B L F I A T E Z C O L L A G E I E U O Z
C P M C S T G X O M X Y A I I M T C I R
M H P B E M Y E P L G Q P T O P E Q L I
C O A R T D E C O R G R T F L R P E P E
Q T I R W Y U M K B E M A U C E O C A Y
V O N D C M Z H V T Y S C F Z S P Z I G
D R T D G O C U S R K S S G F S A Q N U
W E B U Q T A A E Z V G S I T I R I T K
M A R D E W M L N A U W S J O O T N U T
A L U K D I L H G V T B B Y V N M I S E
R I S P L A T T E R A N H V I I I C H R
C S H K G B N R D Z J S G A N S L S W L
W M U S C A L L I G R A P H Y M M J T S
```

OIL PAINT   COLLAGE   POP ART   MASTERPIECE   GRAFFITI   GALLERY ABSTRACT

PAINTING   CALLIGRAPHY   PORTRAIT   ART DECO   SURREALISM   IMPRESSIONISM

SCULPTURE   PHOTOREALISM   PALETTE KNIFE   EXPRESSIONIST   RENAISSANCE

CLAY   CHARCOAL   CANVAS   SKETCH   SPLATTER   PAINTBRUSH   CUBISM

Cryptogram

Using the clues, solve the puzzle to reveal an activity a retiree might do.

1. S
2.
3.
4.
5.
6.
7.
8. M
9.
10.
11.
12.
13.
14.
15.
16.
17.
18.

Guess these foods to solve the puzzle.

1. Liquid comfort in a bowl?

2. Stacked fast food.

3. This dessert is as American as it gets.

4. Rump, round, or sirloin is perfect for this meal.

5. They can be poached or fried.

6. Burger's sidekick?

7. The star of guacamole.

8. This is often eaten with gravy.

9. U.S. state known for potato production.

10. Cuts from young sheep?

11. Probiotic-rich snack.

12. College student's instant meal?

13. Creamy holiday beverage.

14. Crescent-shaped nuts.

15. A scoop that may cause brain freeze?

16. Italy's cheesy gift to the world?

17. This is considered a delicacy by the French.

18. Popular pizza topping.

Crossword

How much do you remember about the Olympics? Use the clues to solve to puzzle.

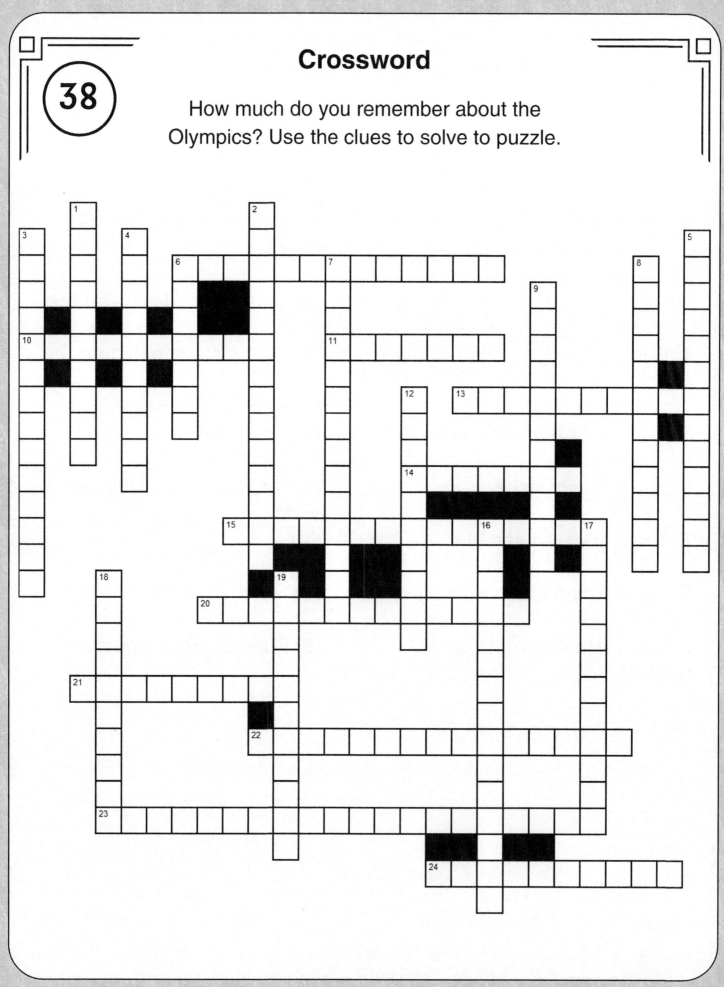

Across

6. Sport introduced at 2020 Games.

10. Comaneci's score?

11. Wenlock and Vinicius are two of these.

13. The only animal sport at the Games.

14. Stones and brooms are needed for this sport.

15. Podium moments during the Games?

20. Harding and Kerrigan's sport.

21. Gretzky's sport.

22. Bolt is no stranger to setting these.

23. Aquatic choreography in harmony?

24. Five-event trial.

Down

1. Celebratory run after a win.

2. Patriotic tune for medal winners?

3. The rulebook of the Games.

4. This sport is all about spikes and digs.

5. Kipchoge's sport.

6. Badminton equipment.

7. Athletes' temporary home during the Games.

8. Ali lit this at the 1996 Games.

9. China dominates in this ball-and-racket sport.

12. Fiery journey to the host city?

16. The grand kickoff?

17. Shaun White's sport.

18. Athens, London and Paris, for example.

19. Shortened version of Lomu and Dupont's sport?

Word Builder

Can you put these letter groups together to form
10-letter words associated with art?

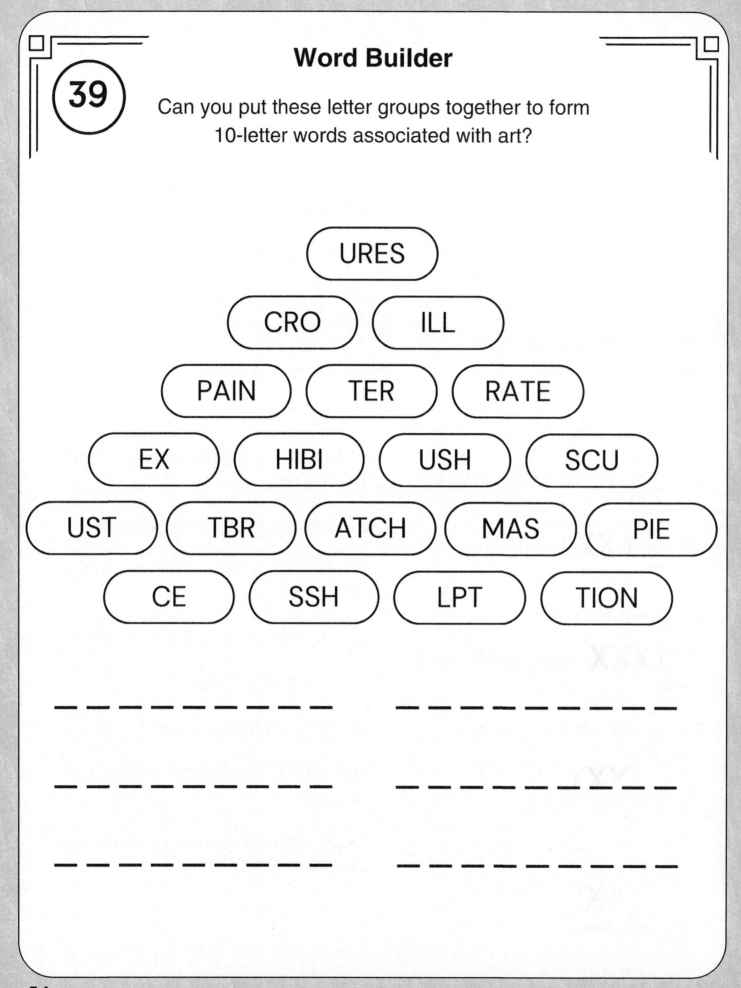

URES

CRO   ILL

PAIN   TER   RATE

EX   HIBI   USH   SCU

UST   TBR   ATCH   MAS   PIE

CE   SSH   LPT   TION

_ _ _ _ _ _ _ _ _ _   _ _ _ _ _ _ _ _ _ _

_ _ _ _ _ _ _ _ _ _   _ _ _ _ _ _ _ _ _ _

_ _ _ _ _ _ _ _ _ _   _ _ _ _ _ _ _ _ _ _

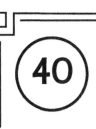

Roman Numerals Calculations

How well do you know the Roman numerals?
Calculate the value of each set of numerals
below.

A.   C – LIX   =

B.   IV × XII   =

C.   LXXXVIII ÷ IV   =

D.   (XXX + XXV) – X   =

E.   XXXIX + XLII   =

F.   LXXIII – XXXVI   =

World Cuisine

Match the countries to their national dishes.

PAELLA	ITALY
RAGU ALLA BOLOGNESE	CHINA
JOLLOF RICE	GERMANY
POUTINE	ICELAND
MOUSSAKA	SPAIN
PEKING DUCK	GHANA
HAGGIS	GREECE
HÁKARL	NIGERIA
SAUERBRATEN	SCOTLAND
FUFU	CANADA

70s and 80s Sitcoms

42

Find your favorite TV comedies of the 70s and 80s in the grid below.

```
F A W L T Y T O W E R S F R S P F Q B G
G A M G G M A U D E B L A C K A D D E R
J T M X A I X M R N I G H T C O U R T C
N H S I L N I E R W T P D K M X D A H H
H E A N L D F U L L H O U S E Q O W R S
C F N T I Y S G S F E K S E Z B P U E T
X A F H N O M A N G O M T E S G M E H
Z C O E T U G A P H O B P V O I I D S E
I T R O H R M T T Z L W O T V T K H C Y
E S D D E L Q R G T D L J H D P K A O O
I O A D F A F C H E E R S O A B B P M U
S F N C A N D W C H N R O O B X L P P N
J L D O M G P I T A G G S O K G U Y A G
R I S U I U L Q R B I O W M V V E D N O
E F O P L A A D J V R C L Z O Y J A Y N
G E N L Y G L Z X A L L O A L L O Y K E
M T H E J E F F E R S O N S F X D S E S
```

ALLO ALLO   FAWLTY TOWERS   BLACKADDER   SANFORD AND SON   SNOW JOB

FAMILY MATTERS   GOOD TIMES   THE YOUNG ONES   MIND YOUR LANGUAGE

CHEERS   THREE'S COMPANY   NIGHT COURT   ALICE   HAPPY DAYS

ALL IN THE FAMILY   ALF   THE LOVE BOAT   FULL HOUSE   THE FACTS OF LIFE

THE ODD COUPLE   SOAP   TAXI   MAUDE   THE JEFFERSONS

Unscramble the Words

Unscramble these words associated with fishing.

FAYSRIHC   _ _ _ _ _ _ _ _

FIGFISHLYN   _ _ _ _ _ _ _ _ _ _

GANGILN   _ _ _ _ _ _ _

NMSOLA   _ _ _ _ _ _

SERFWREATH   _ _ _ _ _ _ _ _ _ _

SCAUNCRATE   _ _ _ _ _ _ _ _ _ _

EBBORB   _ _ _ _ _ _

IRKSEN   _ _ _ _ _ _

"I'm not just retiring from the company, I'm also retiring from my stress, my commute, my alarm clock, and my iron."

Hartman Jule

44

Guess the thing, event, or person associated
with the group of 3 words

A

ACUTE

OBTUSE

REFLEX

....

B

SPEAR

FLY

NET

....

C

ROSÉ

FORTIFIED

SPARKLING

....

D

JACK DORSEY

REID HOFFMAN

LARRY PAGE

....

E

GEORGE ELIOT

JRR TOLKIEN

ZADIE SMITH

....

Roman Numerals Calculations

How well do you know the Roman numerals?
Calculate the value of each set of numerals
below.

A   L – X   =

B   IX x II   =

C   XC / III   =

D   C – XXV   =

E   XL + XV   =

F   VI x IV   =

Trivia

Test your knowledge of popular hobbies!

1. What popular hobby involves growing vegetables?
a) Knitting
b) Gardening
c) Fishing
d) Painting

2. What activity involves creating patterns with yarn?
a) Birdwatching
b) Cooking
c) Crochet
d) Hiking

3. What pastime does a bibliophile love?
a) Cooking
b) Playing tennis
c) Swimming
d) Reading

4. Which hobby involves making furniture?
a) Cycling
b) Woodworking
c) Playing chess
d) Gardening

5. What activity would you use bobbers and lures for?
a) Pottery
b) Painting
c) Photography
d) Fishing

6. What activity involves making bouquets?
a) Flower arranging
b) Skateboarding
c) Sculpting
d) Running

7. You would use a kiln for which activity?
a) Pottery
b) Dancing
c) Surfing
d) Bowling

8. What relaxing hobby involves envelopes?
a) Ice skating
b) Cycling
c) Stamp collecting
d) Jogging

9. Which popular hobby involves making quilts?
a) Camping
b) Playing cards
c) Sewing
d) Scuba diving

10. What activity involves organizing and storing old family photos?
a) Gardening
b) Fishing
c) Scrapbooking
d) Running

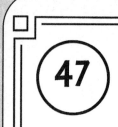

Decrypt the historical events using
the key below.

A	B	C	D	E	F	G	H	I	J	K	L	M
21	23	4	17	5	20	12	8	26	6	9	15	1

N	O	P	Q	R	S	T	U	V	W	X	Y	Z
7	25	24	16	10	19	18	13	3	11	22	14	2

A

| 15 | 21 | 13 | 7 | 4 | 8 | | 25 | 20 | | 19 | 24 | 13 | 18 | 7 | 26 | 9 |

B

| 26 | 7 | 3 | 5 | 7 | 18 | 26 | 25 | 7 | | 25 | 20 | | 18 | 8 | 5 |

| 26 | 7 | 18 | 5 | 10 | 7 | 5 | 18 |

C

| 4 | 8 | 5 | 10 | 7 | 23 | 25 | 14 | 15 | | 17 | 26 | 19 | 21 | 19 | 18 | 5 | 10 |

48

Decrypt the names of famous poets
using the key below.

A	B	C	D	E	F	G	H	I	J	K	L	M
21	23	4	17	5	20	12	8	26	6	9	15	1

N	O	P	Q	R	S	T	U	V	W	X	Y	Z
7	25	24	16	10	19	18	13	3	11	22	14	2

(A)

| 1 | 21 | 14 | 21 | | 21 | 7 | 12 | 5 | 15 | 25 | 13 |

(B)

| 10 | 25 | 23 | 5 | 10 | 18 | | 20 | 10 | 2 | 19 | 18 |

(C)

| 10 | 13 | 1 | 26 |

49

Solve the math problems below.

1. If the cost of living increases by 2% annually and a retiree's annual expenses are currently $40,000, what will their expenses be in 5 years?

_ _ _ _ _ _ _

2. Emily's garden is divided into a vegetable patch, a flower bed, and a herb garden. The vegetable patch is 15 x 10 ft., the flower bed is 12 x 9 ft., and the herb garden is 8 x 7 ft. What is the total area of Emily's garden? (Hint: L(ft) x W(ft) = A ft^2).

_ _ _ _ _ _ _

3. Joe plays 3 rounds of golf each week, with each round taking 4 hours. If he plays for 8 weeks, how many total hours does he spend playing golf?

4. Kelly makes a recipe that requires 2.5 cups of flour per batch, and she plans to make 7 batches, how many cups of flour would she need in total?

_ _ _ _ _ _ _

5. If Shiloh plays bridge twice a week and each game takes 2.5 hours, how many hours will she spend playing bridge in a month (assuming 4 weeks)?

_ _ _ _ _ _ _

Staying Healthy

Find these words related to health and wellness
in the grid below.

```
B O I W R M Z V V E G E T A B I E S U P
L E K U X I M S I I S V N P L A Y B F D
C Y Z U A N S B T S L F U T N T F G S A
S H Y G I E N E A F E X F U V H R C U C
V N O N N R Y M M R E L A X A T I O N T
B Y D L F A E J I U P S L E K N E I S I
I S L I Y L N X N I A G S Y A Q N I C V
C E Q T C S A A S T V I E G M M D P R E
W C F S N I T R C A D R E Z W S P E L
O M U J T X I R H R C O L V T U H X E I
Y M E N T A L H E A L T H W R M I K N F
X E B D H C K X C S E Z Y S F N P U Q E
N U W S I G E C K A S U T X W X S P A S
L R E O Q C G S U P P L E M E N T S O T
B R X D Y D I X P H Y S I C I A N M K Y
F O K A R P Q N E G A A R U Q R R Z I L
E N J T H J C H E A L T H Y F A T S Z E
```

SUPPLEMENTS   SLEEP   VEGETABLES   FRUIT   MINERALS

VITAMINS   EXERCISE   HYGIENE   STRESS   ACTIVE LIFESTYLE

SUNSCREEN   SAUNA   YOGA   ORGANIC   FRESH AIR   CHECK UP

FRIENDSHIPS   MUSCLE MASS   MENTAL HEALTH   PHYSICIAN   WELLNESS

MEDICINE   PLAY   RELAXATION   HEALTHY FATS

Crossword

Use the clues to guess the words associated
with retirement.

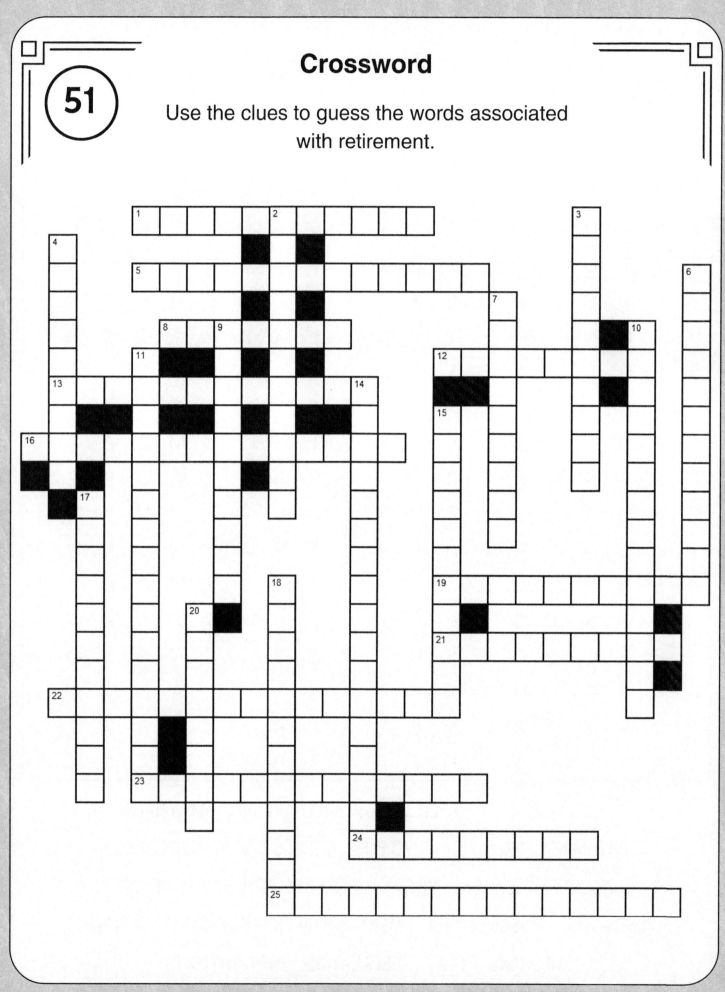

Across

1. Your new familial role, perhaps?

5. Safety net for your loved ones.

8. Passions you can pursue.

12. Type of job for the semi-retired?

13. Hub for social activities for over 65s?

16. Uncle Sam's retirement safety net?

19. Royal Caribbean, for example.

21. Fixed payouts for life.

22. End-of-career celebration?

23. Age at which you stop the daily grind?

24. New career or passion after retirement.

25. Incentives to delay your retirement?

Down

2. Pool of money for retirees?

3. Trading unneeded space for simplicity?

4. A short, fun outing.

6. Holiday nest?

7. A collection of assets.

9. Planned list of adventures?

10. The 65+ year-old club?

11. Expert offering guidance on money matters.

14. Stash for your golden years?

15. The heir to your fortune?

17. Time to enjoy the fruits of your labor.

18. Giving back in your free time.

20. Perks of being a seasoned citizen.

Safe Code

52

Identify the number pattern and replace the blank spaces with the correct digits to unlock the safe.

A

2		12	20
	12	24	
8	24		80

B

3	9	21	
4		28	48
5	15	37	59

C

1	5		25
3		21	
5	15	33	55

D

1	2	4	8
1	3		27
1	4	16	

"You are never too old to set another goal or to dream a new dream."

C. S. Lewis

Number Squares

53

Fill in the boxes to complete the calculations below.

A. (14) + (26) - (8) x (?) = (24)

B. (?) / (5) + (9) x (2) = (27)

C. (36) ? (12) x (2) + (7) = (19)

D. (20) x (3) + (?) / (3) = (75)

E. (81) / (9) ? (14) x (2) = (43)

Guess the Country

54

Test your geography knowledge - identify the countries below!

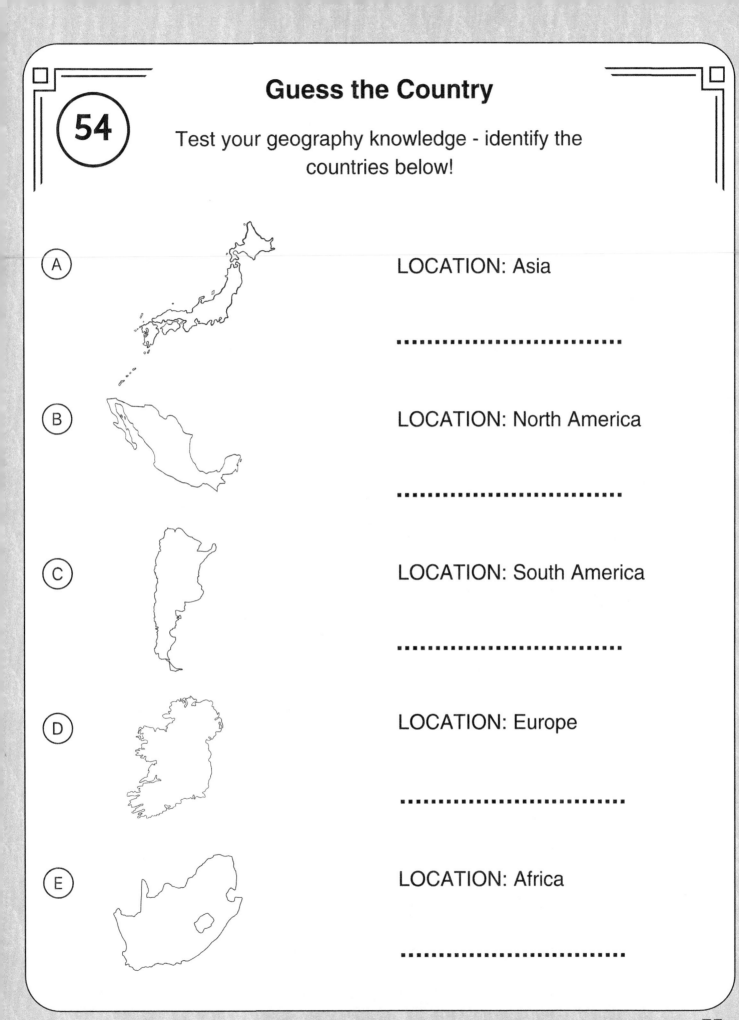

A

LOCATION: Asia

....

B

LOCATION: North America

....

C

LOCATION: South America

....

D

LOCATION: Europe

....

E

LOCATION: Africa

....

Maze

Find your way through this maze!

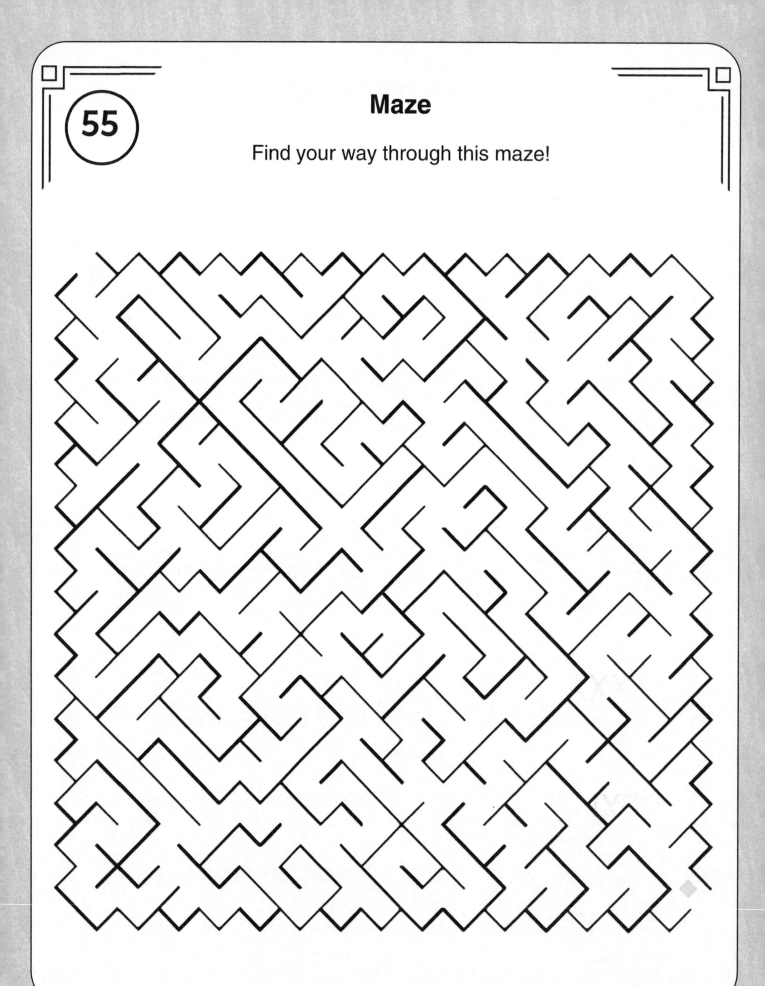

Roman Numerals Calculations

How well do you know the Roman numerals?
Calculate the value of each set of numerals below.

(A) $VIII \times VII$ =

(B) $DCCLXXXIV \div VIII$ =

(C) $(C - XX) + XII$ =

(D) $LXXX + XXVII$ =

(E) $CCXLIV - CLXV$ =

(F) $IX \times VI$ =

Sudoku

Fill each square with a number from 1 to 9 without repeating a number in the vertical or horizontal columns.

Sudoku 13

6		1			9	4		
	8			7	2			
		5	1	6				
				1				
	7		5			8		
			9	4				
			6				9	
9				2		1		7
	1	4				8		

Sudoku 14

4	8		6					5
		2			1			
		1						2
	2							7
		7	8				2	
6								
		9		6			7	
	5			7	4		9	
			1	5		8		4

Sudoku 15

		2					5	
	8				2	1		
	1							9
			9	1			8	5
7					3			
					7		1	2
3		4		5	1	2		
		7		3				
8								

Sudoku 16

4			2	3	8			
							9	
7		3		9				
6		1	9			2		
		2	3	7				4
8			7			9		
			6					8
9	6			4		7		

Unscramble the Words

58

Unscramble these words related to knitting.

CHITSSPLIT   _ _ _ _   _ _ _ _ _ _

ALIEFIRS   _ _ _ _   _ _ _ _

BCEAL   _ _ _ _ _

ALEGELDING   _ _ _ _ _ _ _   _ _ _

FIBNDOF   _ _ _ _   _ _ _

ACSNOT   _ _ _ _   _ _

ENESLED   _ _ _ _ _ _ _

ATCHICKTBS   _ _ _ _   _ _ _ _ _ _

Word Builder

59

Put these letter groups together to form 8-letter names of popular board games.

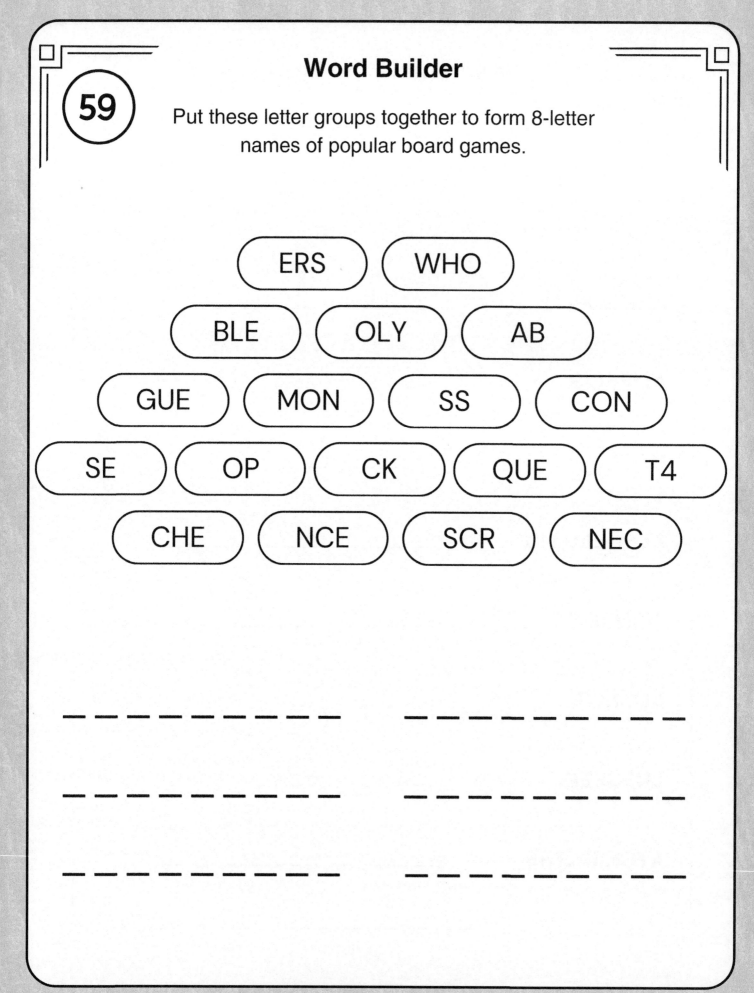

ERS WHO

BLE OLY AB

GUE MON SS CON

SE OP CK QUE T4

CHE NCE SCR NEC

_ _ _ _ _ _ _ _   _ _ _ _ _ _ _ _

_ _ _ _ _ _ _ _   _ _ _ _ _ _ _ _

_ _ _ _ _ _ _ _   _ _ _ _ _ _ _ _

Cryptogram

Decrypt the names of famous animals
using the key below.

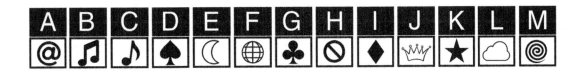

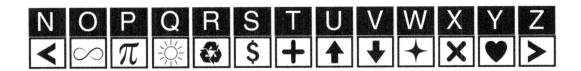

A

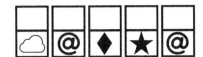

B

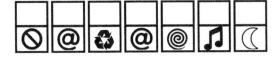

C

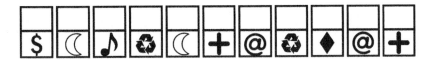

Crossword

How many TV shows of the 70s do you remember? Use the clues to guess the shows.

Across

2. Follow the Time Lord's adventures in this show.

9. Misadventures of a bottle capping duo?

11. Sail along on the MS Pacific Princess in this show.

13. Jim Rockford is a P.I with a knack for trouble.

16. This group supposedly has an airborne circus.

18. Esther and Fred battle it out in this sitcom.

21. JJ, James, Florida, and Willona are in this sitcom.

22. Bionic astronaut?

23. Detective duo aided by "Huggy Bear"?

Down

1. She's in "satin tights fighting for her rights".

3. Crime-fighting trio with a mysterious boss.

4. Ayyyy! Have you seen Richie?

5. "We're movin' on up" with George and Weezy in this show.

6. Musical family touring in a bus?

7. Korean War field hospital comedy-drama.

8. Three roommates navigate life in this sitcom.

10. Hotel run by cantankerous British owner.

11. "Here's the story of a lovely lady..."

12. Lou Ferrigno plays this superhero.

14. Put up with Archie Bunker's antics in this sitcom.

15. Long-running soap set in Weatherfield.

17. Rose, Blanche, Dorothy, and Sophia?

19. Lollipop-sucking detective?

20. Oil tycoon drama set in Texas.

Calculation Questions

Solve the math problems below.

1. Lucas goes fishing and catches an average of 5 fish per hour. If he fishes for 6 hours a day over a weekend (2 days), how many fish would he catch in total?

– – – – – – –

2. Maxine reads 50 pages a day and finishes a 300-page book, how many days will it take her to read 4 books of the same length?

– – – – – – –

3. Abby and Mae plan a road trip covering 1,200 miles in total. If they drive an average of 60 miles per hour and plan to drive for 5 hours each day, how many days will it take to complete the trip?

– – – – – – –

4. Martha knits a scarf that requires 1.5 yards of yarn per foot. If the scarf is 6 feet long, how many yards of yarn does she need?

– – – – – – –

5. If Ken and Paul play a board game that takes 90 minutes per game and they play 4 games in one day, how many hours do they spend playing board games?

– – – – – – –

Learning music

63

Thinking of learning a new instrument? Find these musical words in the grid below.

```
I F Q E G E S B P S T R U M P K I Z F Z
P N J V L E S S O N S R H E E F F B U G
V T R E A Z W D Z Z A H F T R L I R H K
D T R R B N W D C W X Y T R J R O C K V
G U I T A R K D C O O T D O W X T D K V
B C X E P Q X Y L O P H O N E I N R Y E
A L F M T X F L B R H M K O P D M U O K
B A G P I P E S S A O A P M I T Z M P O
I S G O S C A L E P N A R E A T V X C V
K S H Z C V B B N I E D A M N W Y J Y O
R I K S H E E T M U S I C G O R O T E Z
E C K I M P R O V I S A T I O N U M Z P
I A A N C O M P O S I T I O N L Y A E I
R L C U K K A Q N I E L C D R F J J S X
P N D J I R F T R U M P E T W E Q G T A
A W R Q R W T H A F B A K Z S H D G F P
D X Y B Z I K P O F K K T I D O L B O N
```

STRUM   TEMPO   METRONOME   RHYTHM   BAGPIPES   LESSONS   JAZZ

PRACTICE   IMPROVISATION   SHEET MUSIC   SAXOPHONE

MELODY   XYLOPHONE   PITCH   COMPOSITION   TRUMPET   DRUM   BAND

CELLO   GUITAR   PIANO   HARMONY   CLASSICAL   SCALE   ROCK

What Goes Where?

Group the words below into the 3 categories given.

Match these languages to their country or region.

Farsi   **Okinawan**   **Castilian**

Kurdish   **Catalan**

Galician   **Tajik**   **Amami**

PERSIA   JAPAN   SPAIN

"When you retire, you switch bosses - from the one who hired you to the one who married you."

Gene Perret

Word Association

Guess the thing, event, or person associated
with the group of 3 words

A

DIYAS

GARLANDS

CURRY

....

B

NAVAGIO

BONDI

WAILOALOA

....

C

SHETLAND

CONNEMARA

ANADOLU

....

D

CLAM

SNAIL

MUSSEL

....

E

CARAMBOLA

RAMBUTAN

PITAYA

....

Billiard Balls

Fill in the boxes to complete the calculations below.

(A)  + 25 / 5 = 19

(B) 48 ? 6 - 7 = 1

(C) 36 ? 8 X 2 = 20

(D) 50 / ? + 9 = 14

(E) 72 - 18 / ? = 66

Cryptogram

Decrypt the names of famous
activists using the key below.

A	B	C	D	E	F	G	H	I	J	K	L	M
21	23	4	17	5	20	12	8	26	6	9	15	1

N	O	P	Q	R	S	T	U	V	W	X	Y	Z
7	25	24	16	10	19	18	13	3	11	22	14	2

A

1	21	15	21	15	21		14	25	13	19	21	20	2	21	26

B

11	5	23		17	13		23	25	26	19

C

6	21	7	5		20	25	7	17	21

Word Association

Guess the thing, event, or person associated
with the group of 3 words

A
GIGHA
LEWIS AND HARRIS
NORTH UIST

....

B
EXTRA
ECLIPSE
BIG RED

....

C
TORNADO
EMERALD CITY
YELLOW BRICK ROAD

....

D
SMOOTH
LATIN
BEBOP

....

E
GROAN
WHIMPER
MUMBLE

....

Maze

(69)

Find your way through this maze!

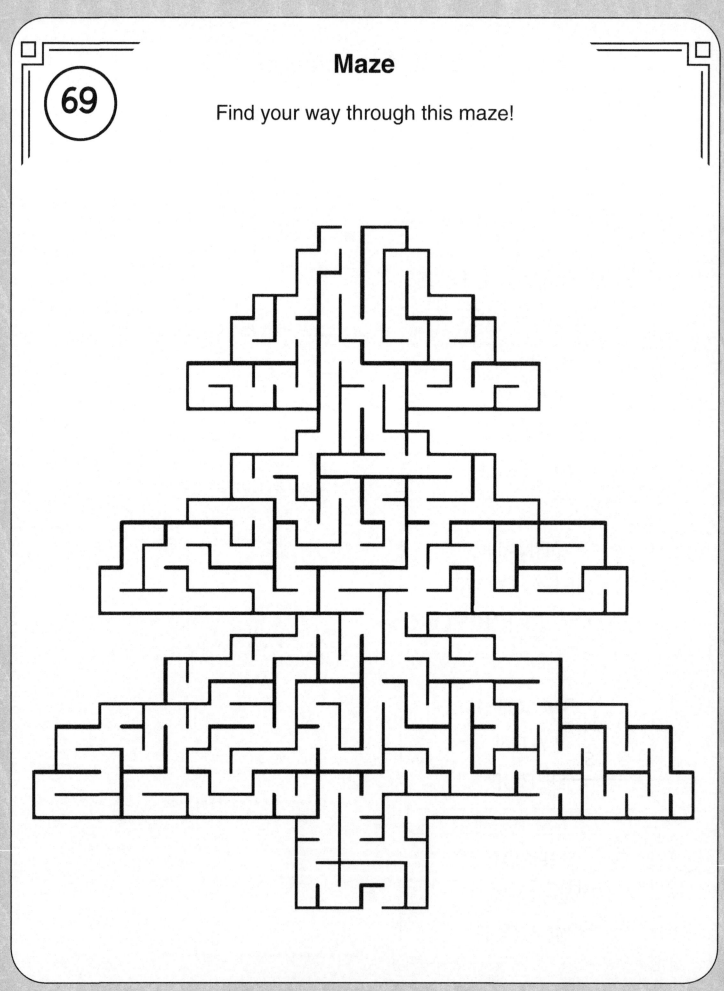

Fashion Trends

Remember these fashion trends? Find them in the grid below.

```
S O J P O W E R S U I T M D Z C W X F A
S C E W S K I N N Y J E A N S A F L I V
G P L E G H S P A N D E X M T T N P N I
V N L P V P O N C H O S I B I E Y E G A
U W Y A I X S U Q Y R Z S A B Y H A E T
B B S T T U H M L E F M K G I E A S R O
R A A C I F D O F D O J I G K G W A L R
Y L N H R B O A T T E M R Y I L A N E S
B L D W E S O R T P Q R T J N A I T S U
M E A O N L A O M R A U P E I S I B S N
W T L R C K B M F S A N T A T S A L G G
H F S K Q L Z F B E H C T N D E N O L L
W L E J L Q T Y P D Q O K S D S S U O A
X A F E D O R A W U V X E S Q D H S V S
R T B A L E G W A R M E R S U K I E E S
E S Q N D D Y K Z M I N I S K I R T S E
Z X O S L E A T H E R J A C K E T V T S
```

MINI SKIRT   BAGGY JEANS   BIKINI   TRACKSUIT   LOAFERS   SKINNY JEANS

PEASANT BLOUSE   BELLBOTTOMS   LEG WARMERS   BALLET FLATS   POWER SUIT

FEDORA   PLATFORM SHOES   AVIATOR SUNGLASSES   SPANDEX   HAWAIIAN SHIRT

CAT-EYE GLASSES   JELLY SANDALS   LEATHER JACKET   HOT PANTS   PONCHOS

SHOULDER PADS   PATCH WORK JEANS   MAXI SKIRT   FINGERLESS GLOVES

Trivia

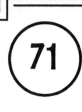

How much do you know about the younger generation?

1. What popular video game is about building and exploring?
a) Fortnite
b) Minecraft
c) Among Us
d) Roblox

2. Which animated movie features characters named Elsa and Anna?
a) Frozen
b) Toy Story
c) Moana
d) Zootopia

3. What school does Harry Potter and friends attend?
a) Hogwarts
b) Neverland
c) Narnia
d) Middle-earth

4. Who is the lead character in the "Paw Patrol" series?
a) Ryder
b) Chase
c) Marshall
d) Rubble

5. Which toy line features Optimus Prime and Bumblebee?
a) Transformers
b) Power Rangers
c) Teenage Mutant Ninja Turtles
d) Hot Wheels

6. What popular app involves creating short videos with music?
a) Instagram
b) Snapchat
c) TikTok
d) Facebook

7. What world is Pokémon set in?
a) Narnia
b) Alagaësia
c) Middle-earth
d) Pokémon World

8. Which popular book series is about a young wizard?
a) Percy Jackson
b) Harry Potter
c) The Hunger Games
d) Diary of a Wimpy Kid

9. What kind of animal is the main character in "Peppa Pig"?
a) Pig
b) Rabbit
c) Dog
d) Cat

10. What is the name of the famous Fortnite dance move?
a) Floss
b) Macarena
c) Twist
d) Slide

Sudoku

Fill each square with a number from 1 to 9 without repeating a number in the vertical or horizontal columns.

Sudoku 17

		9						
			1	5		7		4
	5			8	7			
		3					1	7
2				4		8		
	4			3			2	5
		8			3			
		1	5		4			
			8	2				

Sudoku 18

								3
5		1	7	8				
	2		1			4		
			5					
4				8				
		3	7	1	6			
	3	6						
			3	2	8			
			4	5				2

Sudoku 19

9								
7				9		4		6
		6	3			7	8	
2			6		7		5	
	9	7		3				
		9		2	8			
4	6							
	2	8			5			

Sudoku 20

		1						
3	6				8		9	5
	8	9						7
		6	5	3		7		
			1			3		4
1						6		8
	1	3	4					
4				7				
5	7							6

Word Builder

73

Can you put these letter groups together to form
6-letter words associated with golf?

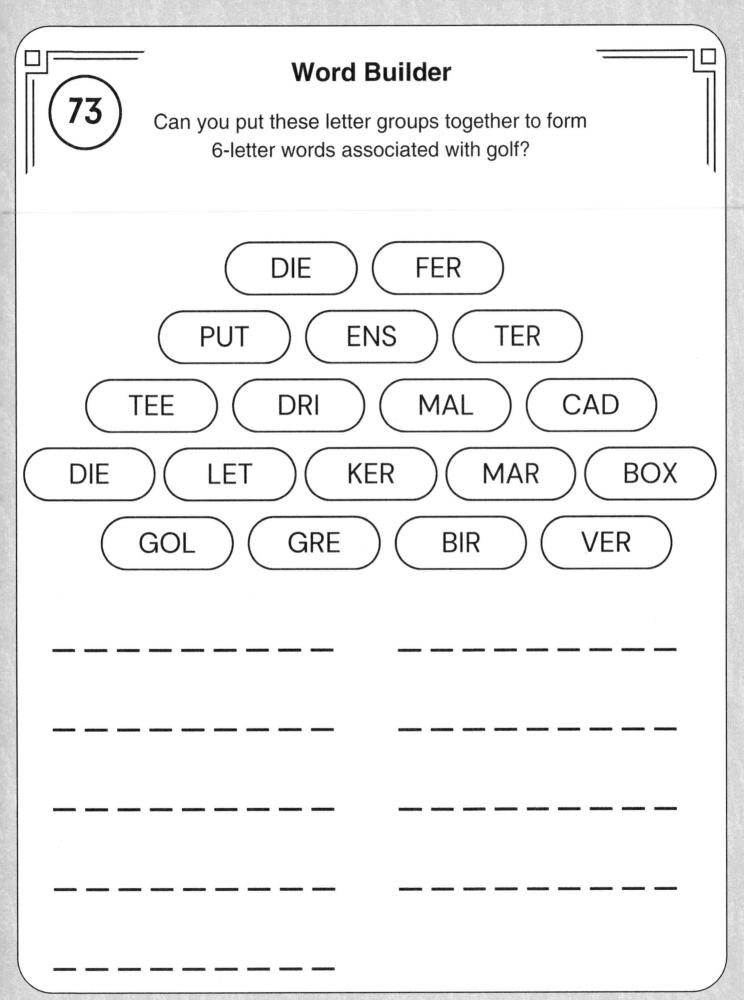

DIE   FER

PUT   ENS   TER

TEE   DRI   MAL   CAD

DIE   LET   KER   MAR   BOX

GOL   GRE   BIR   VER

\- \- \- \- \- \- \- \- \- \-   \- \- \- \- \- \- \- \-

\- \- \- \- \- \- \- \- \- \-   \- \- \- \- \- \- \- \-

\- \- \- \- \- \- \- \- \- \-   \- \- \- \- \- \- \- \-

\- \- \- \- \- \- \- \- \- \-   \- \- \- \- \- \- \- \-

\- \- \- \- \- \- \- \- \- \-

Cryptogram

74

Using the clues, solve the puzzle to reveal a
project your grand kids would love.

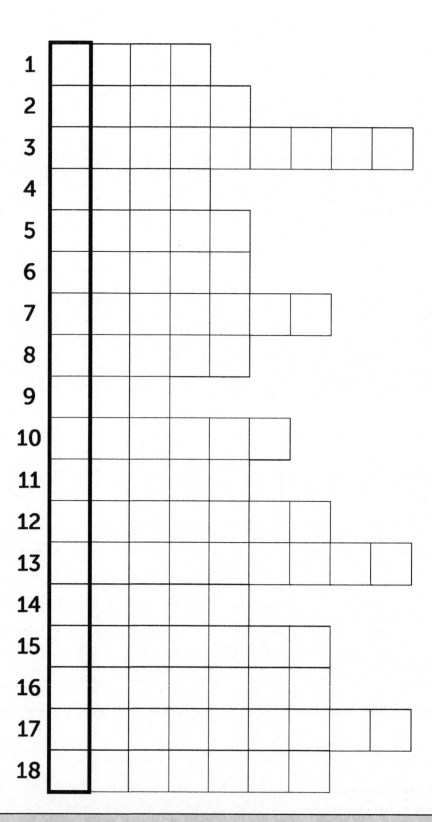

Figure out the answers to these clues!

1. Hardworking pollinators.

2. Queen song, "_____ Pressure".

3. Life, home, or family _____.

4. Mufasa is one.

5. Computer data is stored on this.
.

6. Ebony and _____.

7. Whitney Houston song, "I Have _____".

8. Green TV character made of clay.

9. Main insect in "A Bug's Life".

10. Key veggie in Italian cuisine.

11. Animal that has rabies.

12. Song by Gaye, "Mercy Mercy Me (The _____)"

13. The height of land above sea level.

14. Marge's husband.

15. Animal with 4 hearts?

16. Hawaii's state instrument.

17. Doctor Octopus' nemesis.

18. Peak that Edmund Hillary is known for.

Crossword

Find the names of musicians of the
70s and 80s using the clues below.

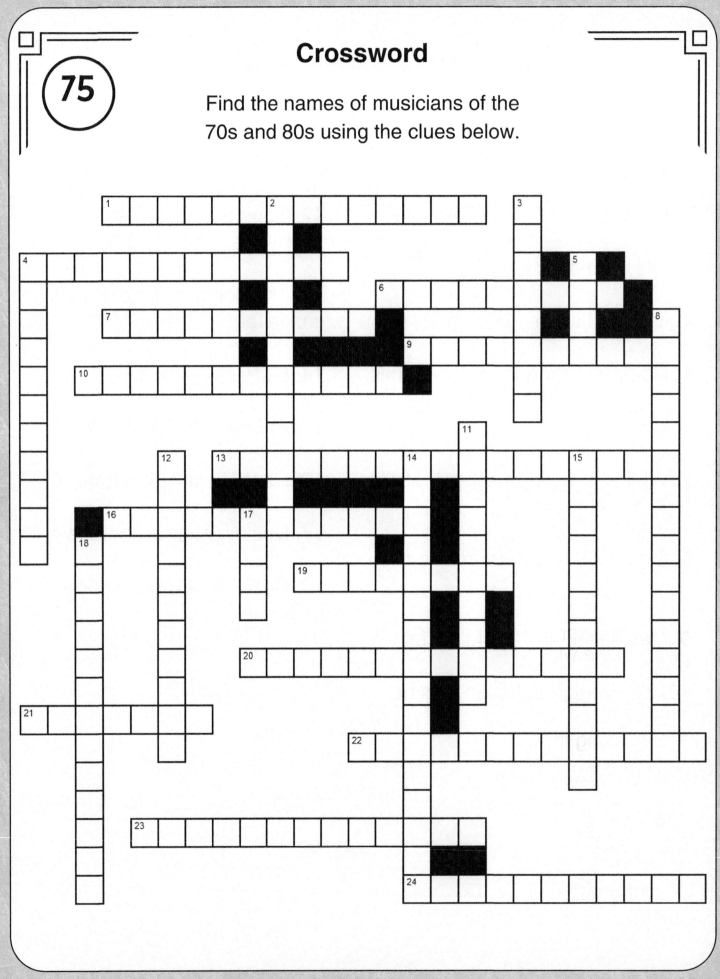

Across

1. The "Queen of Soul".

4. She's looked at life from both sides now.

6. Rocket man, piano man, or both?

7. Formerly, The Quarrymen.

9. He knew about a boy named "Sue".

10. Harmonica-playing musical genius.

13. Folk duo known for "Mrs. Robinson".

16. Boy band with "Good Vibrations"?

19. The answer to this one is blowin' in the wind.

20. Frankie Valli's group.

21. Hitmaking trio of brothers.

22. Bowie's alter ego.

23. Sibling duo known for "Close to You".

24. "Hot Stuff" and Last Dance" singer.

Down

2. Stevie Nicks' group?

3. It's not unusual to love this singer's music.

4. He played the "Star Spangled Banner" at Woodstock.

5. Nile Rodgers' disco band.

8. A rock band…or copies of a popular magazine.

11. Georgia was on his mind.

12. Diana, Mary, and Florence made up this Motown group.

14. "Son of a Preacher Man" singer.

15. Her boots were made for walking.

17. Agnetha, Anni-Frid, Björn, and Benny.

18. They think it's fun to stay at the Y.M.C.A.

Billiard Balls

Fill in the boxes to complete the calculations below.

 20 **?** 2 **-** 15 **=** 25

B 63 **/** **?** **+** 10 **=** 19

C **?** **-** 12 **/** 3 **=** 39

D 80 **/** 8 **?** 6 **=** 16

E 54 **-** **?** **X** 2 **=** 36

"First you forget names; then you forget faces; then you forget to zip up your fly, and then you forget to unzip your fly."

Branch Rickey

77

Solve the math problems below.

1. Jackson develops his photos in sets of 36. If he has 5 sets of photos, and each set costs $8 to develop, how much will he spend in total to develop all the photographs?

_ _ _ _ _ _ _

2. Sarah spends 3 hours painting each day for 5 days a week. How many hours does she spend painting in 6 weeks?

_ _ _ _ _ _ _

3. John spots an average of 12 different bird species per outing. If he goes birdwatching 4 times a month, how many different bird species will he spot in 3 months?

_ _ _ _ _ _ _

4. Emily bakes cookies and uses 3/4 cups of sugar per batch. If she bakes 10 batches in a week, how many cups of sugar will she need in total for 4 weeks?

_ _ _ _ _ _ _

5. Michael plays tennis for 2 hours every Monday, Wednesday, and Friday. How many hours does he play tennis in a month (assuming 4 weeks)?

_ _ _ _ _ _ _

Cryptogram

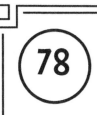

78

Decrypt the names of famous European landmarks using the key below.

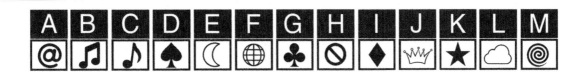

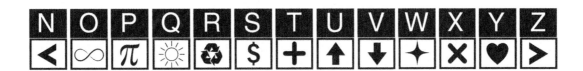

Ⓐ

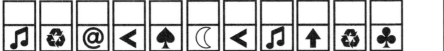 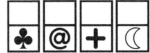

Ⓑ

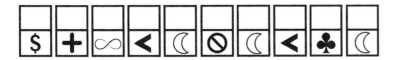

Ⓒ

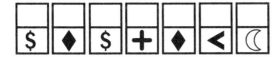 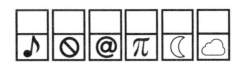

Historic Events

Match the significant event to the year it happened.

OPENING OF DISNEY WORLD	2004
MOON LANDING	1969
LAUNCH OF FACEBOOK	2010
DEATH OF PRINCESS DIANA	1985
CHALLENGER DISASTER	1997
THATCHER BECOMES U.K PM	1971
FALL OF THE BERLIN WALL	1986
LAUNCH OF PLAYSTATION 1	1979
LIVE AID CONCERT	1989
LAUNCH OF THE IPAD	1994

Yoga

80

Find the terms associated with yoga in the grid below.

```
S P I R I T U A L I T Y B N C D T K T U
B C P X X I R G N X O N I R V A N A F Q
B I R Y U D I N S T R U C T O R D T P O
D O A I H Y U S T R E N G T H E U E D Y
N F C B G B R E A T H I N G V O I R Z I
Q H T C B Y D H I Y I O V R K F Z F W T
O I I P A H O O A E I V U R P F S U Y C
E N C O L C N G W T I Y O G A M A T A S
N D I S A V A S A N A W Y I J J A M P E
A U N E N H F T F C W F I T N E S S G N
B I G S C Z I P C H L A L J J I A F F X
K S T M E D G O S O A A R E H D N U P I
D M O V E M E N T S W S S D X B A X M K
Z D A M U S C L E S W P D S D I J Y F S
Z C H A K R A N W E Y U U M E O B P N P
X C B L A E L P Y J B J Y S V S G L Z K
C F A U J N S T R E T C H I N G A V E S
```

MEDITATION   SAVASANA   NIRVANA   STRETCHING   FITNESS   POSES

PRACTICING   YOGA MAT   FLEXIBLE   YOGA CLASSES

BUDDHISM   WORKOUT   AYURVEDA   CAT COW   STRENGTH   ASANA

BALANCE   MOVEMENTS   BREATHING   MUSCLES   HINDUISM   CHAKRA

SPIRITUALITY   INSTRUCTOR   DOWNWARD DOG

Roman Numerals Calculations

How well do you know the Roman numerals?
Calculate the value of each set of numerals
below.

(A)   L – XX   =

(B)   VI x III   =

(C)   LXXX / IV   =

(D)   C – XL   =

(E)   XII + IX   =

(F)   XXV + XV   =

Word Association

Guess the thing, event, or person associated
with the group of 3 words

A
MERCURY
APOLLO
ATHENA

....

B
MARPLE
POIROT
HOLMES

....

C
PIROUETTE
WORM
MOONWALK

....

D
WALL STREET
SILICON VALLEY
HOLLYWOOD

....

E
HARPER
BRUCE
SPIKE

....

Crossword

Find the names of musicians of the 80s and 90s using the clues below.

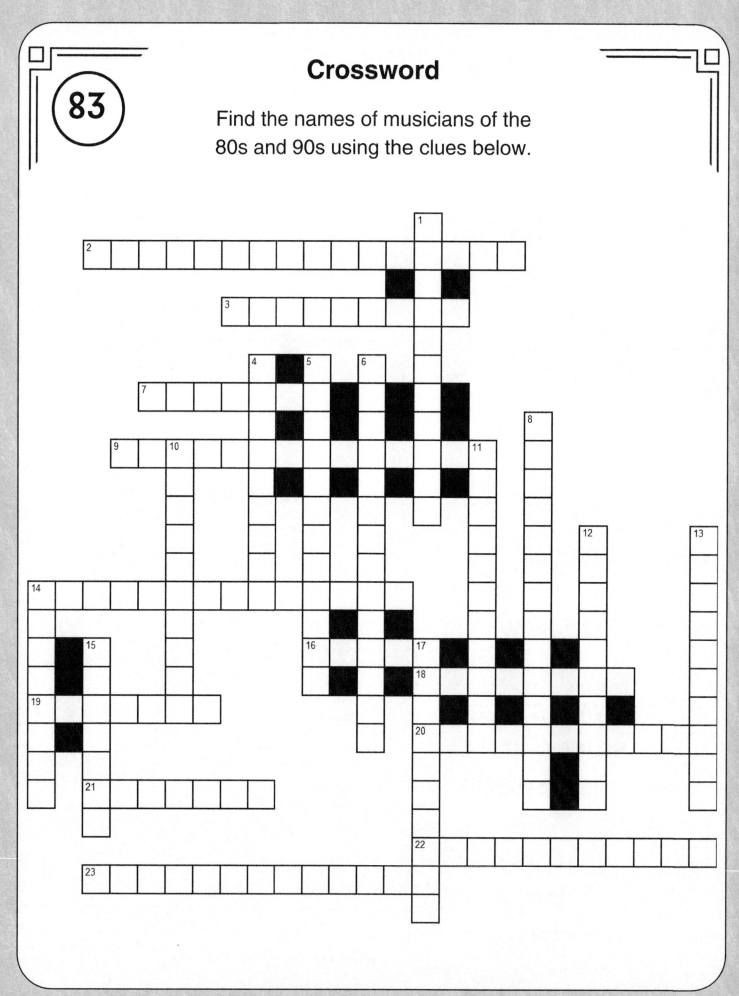

Across

2. "Jagged Little Pill" artist.

3. This group "saw the sign".

7. Rockers who probably smelled like teen spirit.

9. This band wants it that way.

14. The "bad" "man in the mirror"?

16. Band led by Liam Gallagher.

18. Band behind "Alive" and "Jeremy".

19. "Vogue" singer.

20. "Time After Time" singer.

21. Call this band when "the tide is high".

22. "Livin' La Vida Loca" singer.

23. One half of the duo "Wham!"

Down

1. They fought for their right to party.

4. Hip hop duo behind "Push It".

5. She sang "Scream" with her brother.

6. The Voice?

8. Group behind "Hold On".

10. Queen of Power Ballads?

11. Country singer who "feels like a woman".

12. "Summer of '69" singer.

13. "Hungry Like the Wolf" singers.

14. Rapper that you "can't touch".

15. Gwen Stefani's 90s group.

17. Mel B's group.

Safe Code

84

Identify the number pattern and replace the blank spaces with the correct digits to unlock the safe.

A

1	4	9	
2	8		32
3	27	48	

B

2	5		11
	8	12	16
6		18	

C

1		5	7
2	6	10	14
4	12		28

D

1	3	7	
2		12	20
5	15	29	

Unscramble the Words

Unscramble these words associated with spirituality.

ANETTIMIDO   _ _ _ _ _ _ _ _ _

ACEDRS   _ _ _ _ _

IEINVD   _ _ _ _ _ _

LARRUPUNSEAT   _ _ _ _ _ _ _ _ _ _ _

OPSWHIR   _ _ _ _ _ _ _

GAOLSRYOT   _ _ _ _ _ _ _ _ _

CREPTURIS   _ _ _ _ _ _ _ _

ENHEVA   _ _ _ _ _ _

Trivia

How much do you remember about fashion in the 70s?

1. What shoes became popular in the 70s?
a) Flip flops
b) Platform shoes
c) Sandals
d) Ballet flats

2. Which fabric was widely used in 70s bell-bottoms?
a) Denim
b) Silk
c) Velvet
d) Leather

3. What style of pants flared out at the lower legs?
a) Bell-bottoms
b) Skinny jeans
c) Cargo pants
d) Capri pants

4. Which hairstyle did John Travolta wear in Saturday Night Fever?
a) Pompadour
b) Shag
c) Afro
d) Mullet

5. What type of hat did many people wear during the 70s?
a) Bucket hat
b) Fedora
c) Beanie
d) Newsboy cap

6. What was a popular type of women's wear in the 70s?
a) Maxi dress
b) Flannel shirt
c) Pencil skirt
d) Slip dress

7. Which accessory was often worn as a headband?
a) Bandana
b) Scarf
c) Belt
d) Bracelet

8. What type of jacket was popular among men in the 70s?
a) Leather jacket
b) Bomber jacket
c) Trench coat
d) Denim jacket

9. What was a popular women's footwear option in the 70s?
a) Dr. Martens
b) Flip flops
c) Clogs
d) Sneakers

10. What type of collar was trendy on 70s shirts?
a) Turtle neck
b) Peter Pan collar
c) Wide collar
d) Mandarin collar

What Goes Where?

87

Group the words below into the 3 categories given.

Match these cities to their country.

Cologne   **Dijon**   **Salvador**

Strasbourg   **Frankfurt**

Dresden   **Grenoble**   **Belo Horizonte**

GERMANY   FRANCE   BRAZIL

"Dare to live the life you have dreamed for yourself. Go forward and make your dreams come true."

Ralph Waldo Emerson

Maze

(88)

Find your way through this maze!

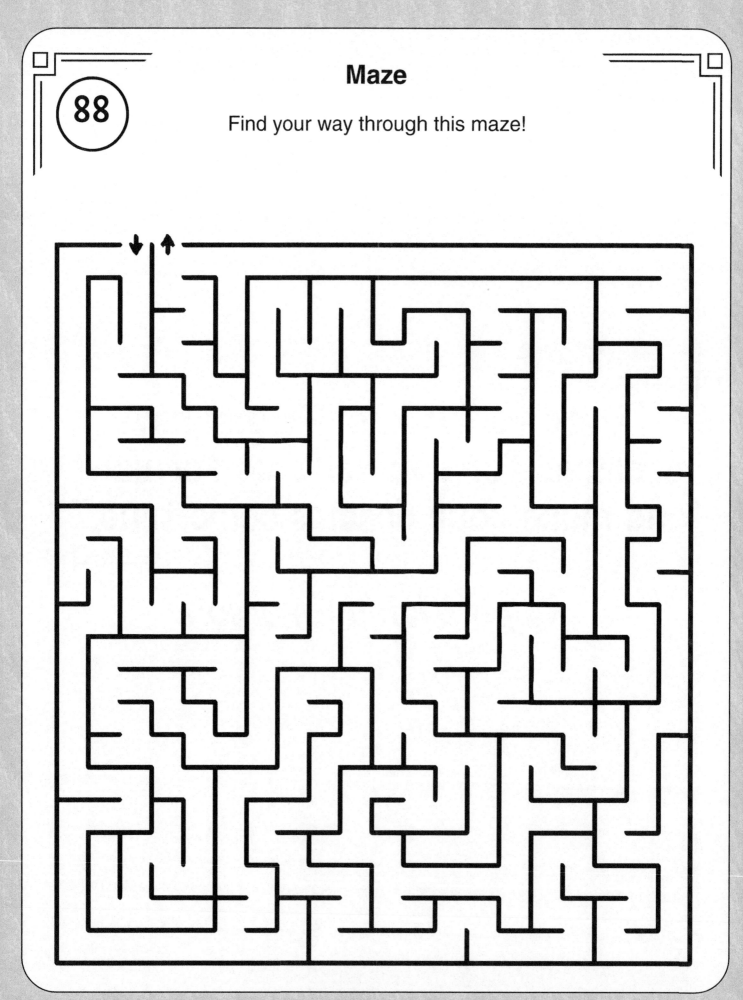

World Leaders

Find leaders of the ancient and modern world in
the grid below.

```
M M G S O D C M F M Y A L E X A N D E R
R K S E G H B I Z C D R Z D Y G S C T T
Z J A D N J V Z D L L D H Z L Q O K F L
Q A S C E G K R A M S E S G B X A M D X
V D C A H G H J A W O R O F P S Z L R K
C Y R U S U A I F J M N V P E L O W O L
O B U A I B R U S K R L T I A O M A O M
X O O I T O W C L K E S Z V R T E T S N
M F G L T S Z H H L H N H X S C R N E A
E E L C I B Z U P I E A N I O D K A V N
U J I F N V M V D M L I N E N R E P E J
L V N J G Q A Q R A D L P O D Z L O L Q
Z J C G B I D R M N H W X B N Y O L T H
S P O S U I L U A D B M N A Q B O E J N
X H L L L I O H J E F F E R S O N O P L
Z L N J L U G K I L C I O M E L O N I T
P J R W R I E T H A T C H E R W O B C Y
```

DE GAULLE   J. F. KENNEDY   CHURCHILL   GHANDI   SITTING BULL

F.D. ROOSEVELT   NAPOLEON   MENZIES   SHINZO   GENGHIS KHAN

RAMSES   CLEOPATRA   ARDERN   VICTORIA   L. B. PEARSON

MANDELA   MELONI   MERKEL   CYRUS   ALEXANDER

THATCHER   BOLÍVAR   LINCOLN   JEFFERSON   MAO

Sudoku

90

Fill each square with a number from 1 to 9 without repeating a number in the vertical or horizontal columns.

Sudoku 21

8			6	5	1	9		3
		6	7			1		
								8
		5		7		8	2	1
						7		6
1		8	5		2		3	7
2	3					5		
					3		8	

Sudoku 22

						7		
9			2					
	8						9	5
				6		8		
			7					
	2	9	5					3
			7			8		
8	5							2
	3	2	9			1		

Sudoku 23

5	4	3	2					
		6	3					
			8		7			
				2	4	8		
			5	8		3	9	
	8	4			3	6	7	
	6					9		
9								
		5	4			8		

Sudoku 24

	2	1	8			5	7	
4								1
	3							
			5	3		7		2
	1						9	
7			2	1			8	
		9					3	8
	7					9		
				1	9	4		

What Goes Where?

Group the words below into the 3 categories given.

Match these vehicles to their manufacturer.

Ranger   Beetle   Silverado

Golf   Thunderbird

Mustang   Corvette   Transporter

FORD   CHEVROLET   VOLKSWAGEN

Cryptogram

Using the clues, solve the puzzle to reveal an
activity a retiree might love.

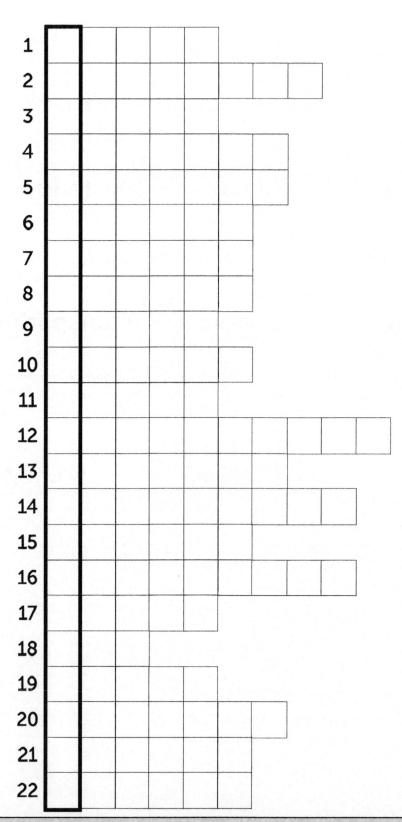

1. South American camelid.

2. Type of animal Dr. Seuss' "Horton" is.

3. Gala or Honeycrisp?

4. Toronto's NBA team.

5. 60's actress "Wood".

6. Tropical lizard

7. Force is measured in this.

8. Sesame Street's incompetent waiter?

9. Sugar substitute from a succulent plant.

10. Idea or belief.

11. Original owner of Graceland

12. Caribbean cricket team.

13. Against the law.

14. Peter Pan's world.

15. Hardly.

16. Film director known for gore.

17. Lucy Ricardo's husband.

18. Popular MMA organization.

19. Sweet fleshy tropical fruit.

20. Barium or Carbon, for example.

21. Novice

22. America's Got _____

Guess the thing, event, or person associated
with the group of 3 words

A ALEXANDER FLEMING
JONAS SALK
EDWARD JENNER

....

B HANDY
GENTLE
NOBLE

....

C POISON DART
GLASS
TREE

....

D GUERNICA
WATER LILIES
STARRY NIGHT

....

E PACIFIC CREST
APPALACHIAN
CONTINENTAL DIVIDE

....

What Goes Where?

94

Group the words below into the 3
categories given.

Match the ancient civilizations to the continent.

Ancient Egypt	**Aztec**	**Maya**
Aksum	**Qin dynasty**	
Olmec	**Harappa**	**Kush**

AFRICA THE AMERICAS ASIA

95

This puzzle is all about hobbies! Use the clues to help you fill in the squares.

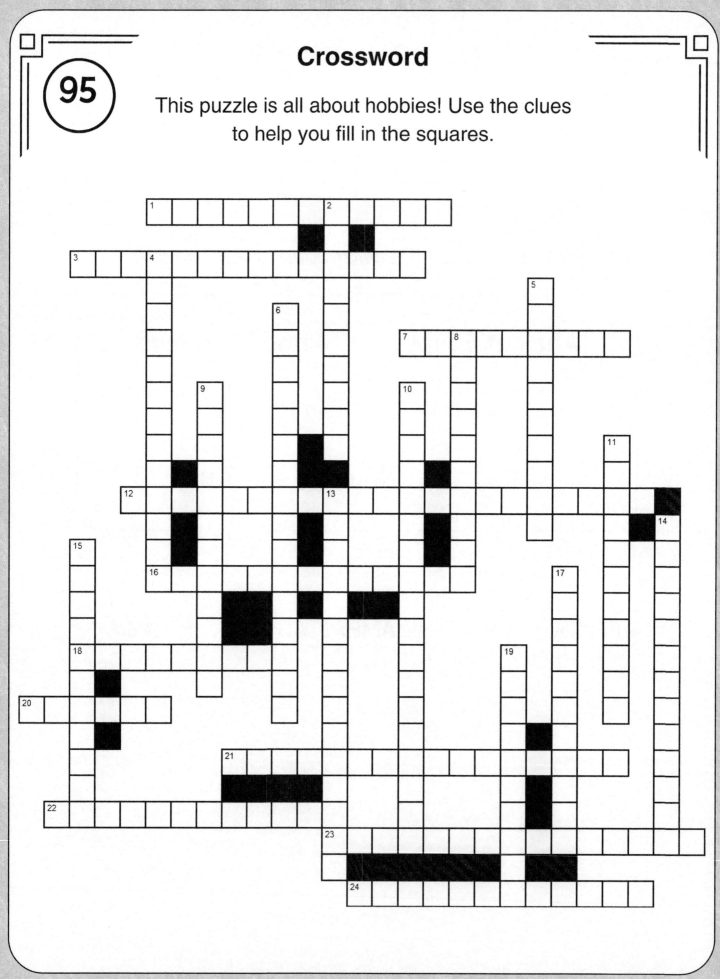

Across

1. It's all about strikes and spares here.

3. Cozy creation from scraps of fabric.

7. Angler's toolbox.

12. Natural way of keeping garden pests away.

16. Hobby involving tracking locomotives.

18. Golfer's dream shot on a par three.

20. Artist's painting surface.

21. Statistic that keeps baseball pitchers on their toes.

22. Searching shorelines for treasures?

23. Keeps adventurers' thirst at bay.

24. Annie Leibovitz's profession.

Down

2. Fish farming and gardening combination.

4. Eco-friendly restroom for campers.

5. Tending to hives?

6. You'll want to use this if you're writing novels.

8. You'll need a hook and yarn loops for this hobby.

9. Hobby involving wax and wicks.

10. Icing sugar.

11. Crafty hobby involving timber.

13. Liquor measurement.

14. A genealogy necessity?

15. A potter's creation.

17. Hobby involving miniature railroads.

19. Perfect time to capture the sunrise or sunset.

Word Builder

Put these letter groups together to form 6-letter names of 80s movie stars.

NOR · KEN · EEP · WEA · INO · RIS · TIS · ISE · CUR · SEA · PAC · SNI · STR · GAL · CRU · WAL · VER · PES

_ _ _ _ _ _   _ _ _ _ _ _

_ _ _ _ _ _   _ _ _ _ _ _

_ _ _ _ _ _   _ _ _ _ _ _

_ _ _ _ _ _   _ _ _ _ _ _

_ _ _ _ _ _

"Some of the best memories are made in flip flops."

Kellie Elmore

Winter Sports

97

Find these cool winter sports in the grid below.

```
E F R E E S T Y L E S K I I N G G H D N
R I N K B A N D Y Y K M F O R N S E O C
E G T W I C E F I S H I N G I G L K G Z
K U O G C Y U N Z H L Y V P B S O C S E
F R B J E R N R P H R A M I B B P I L A
F E O G S Q R V L T F U L O Y R E C E L
M S G A K N E Z F I J E B O Y O S E D P
X K G I A I O X T I N O I G M O T B R I
L A A L T V G W K H C G A V X M Y L A N
D T N M I X E S K E L E T O N B L O C E
X I I F N T T O C I T T H J L A E C I S
U N N E G X D Y B L T T L O B L E K N K
H G G J Y U Z U E W O I O K C L M I G I
J U S P E E D S K A T I N G A K I N N I
L H S N O W M O B I L I N G U H E G Z N
F D U S N O W B O A R D I N G F E Y Z G
F U Q O I C E C L I M B I N G R I G K D
```

ICE SKATING   BOBSLED   TOBOGGANING   FREESTYLE SKIING   SNOWKITING

BIATHLON   LUGE   FIGURE SKATING   CURLING   SNOWBOARDING

SPEED SKATING   SKI JUMPING   SNOWMOBILING   ICE BLOCKING   RINKBALL

SKELETON   RINK BANDY   ALPINE SKIING   ICE FISHING   ICE CLIMBING

SLOPESTYLE   BROOMBALL   ICE HOCKEY   DOGSLED RACING   SLALOM

Inventions & Inventors

98

Match the iconic invention to the company that created it.

WALKMAN	IBM
GAME BOY	WHAM-O
MACINTOSH	DUPONT
MOBILE PHONE	POLAROID
DIGITAL CAMERA	APPLE
SPANDEX	HASBRO
INSTANT FILM	SONY
FRISBEE	NINTENDO
EASY-BAKE OVEN	KODAK
FLOPPY DISK	MOTOROLA

Number Squares

Fill in the boxes to complete the calculations below.

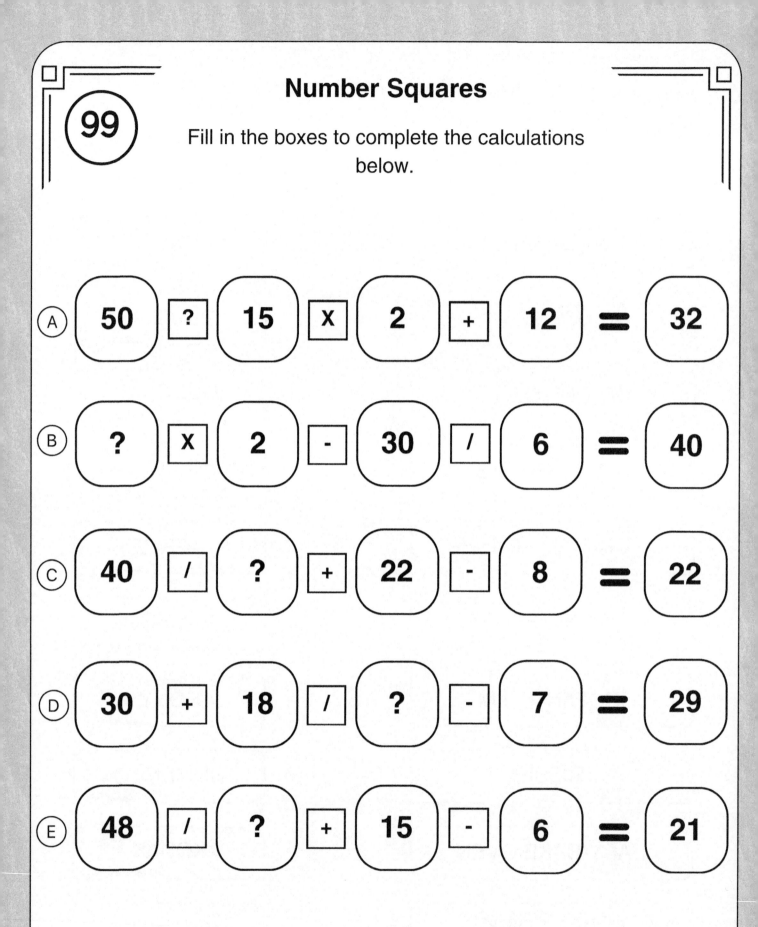

A) 50 [?] 15 [x] 2 [+] 12 = 32

B) ? [x] 2 [-] 30 [/] 6 = 40

C) 40 [/] ? [+] 22 [-] 8 = 22

D) 30 [+] 18 [/] ? [-] 7 = 29

E) 48 [/] ? [+] 15 [-] 6 = 21

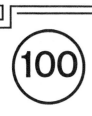

Unscramble the Words

Unscramble these words associated with retirement.

ESMENVTINT   _ _ _ _ _ _ _ _ _

NESPINO   _ _ _ _ _ _ _

ACNERUINS   _ _ _ _ _ _ _ _ _

AVERLT   _ _ _ _ _ _

STASES   _ _ _ _ _ _

AYFLMI   _ _ _ _ _ _

PEATX   _ _ _ _ _

RICEUS   _ _ _ _ _ _ _ _ _

Word Association

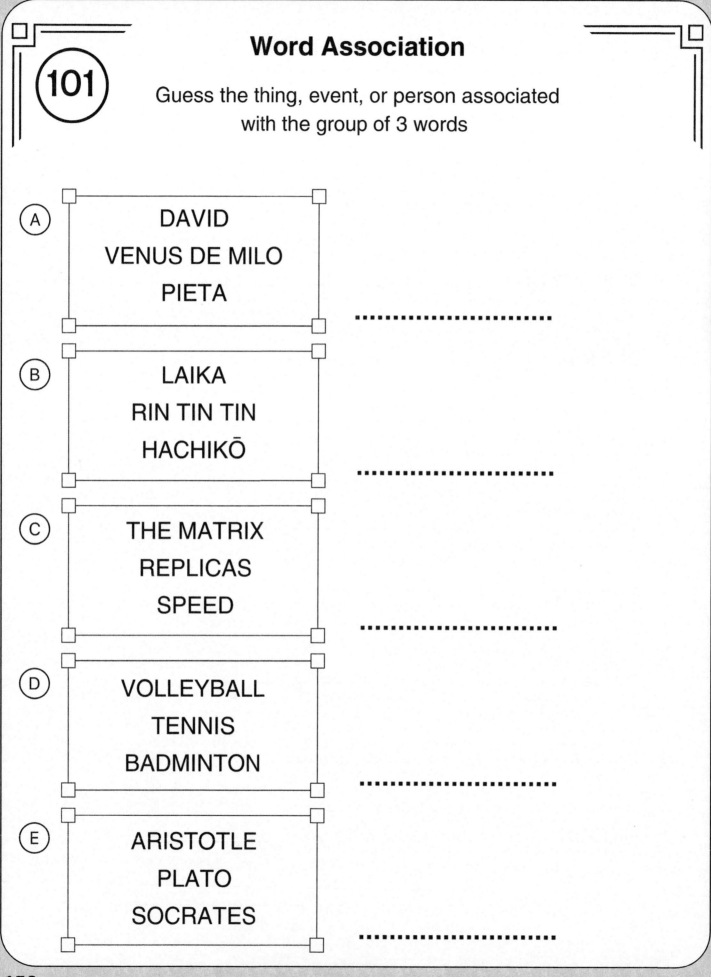

101

Guess the thing, event, or person associated
with the group of 3 words

A

DAVID

VENUS DE MILO

PIETA

....

B

LAIKA

RIN TIN TIN

HACHIKŌ

....

C

THE MATRIX

REPLICAS

SPEED

....

D

VOLLEYBALL

TENNIS

BADMINTON

....

E

ARISTOTLE

PLATO

SOCRATES

....

Congratulations on your retirement and may it be filled with joy and purpose.

Thanks so much for reading and completing my Retirement Activity Book. I really hope you found it both fun and engaging and if so, would kindly ask for a moment of your time to leave a review on Amazon. Reviews help others decide if this is the right book for them so any feedback would be appreciated.

You can leave a review by finding the book on Amazon, then scroll down to the customer review section and click the *'write a customer review'* button.

Thank you.

You can the answers and solutions to all the puzzles on the following pages.

Answers & Solutions

All solutions are labeled by puzzle number not page number.

1

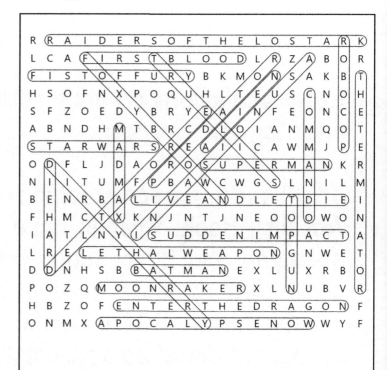

2

A) THE WASHINGTON POST

B) THE GUARDIAN

C) THE TORONTO STAR

3

FRANCE: PERRIER, COGNAC, CHAMPAGNE

MEXICO: MARGARITA, TEQUILA

ITALY: SPRITZ, CAPPUCCINO, ESPRESSO

A) THANKSGIVING

B) WOODSTOCK

C) CAFFEINATED DRINKS

D) DEPARTMENT STORE FOUNDERS

E) COMIC BOOK WRITERS/ARTISTS

Sudoku Solution 1

5	1	7	8	3	4	2	9	6
6	3	8	9	2	1	5	7	4
4	2	9	7	5	6	3	1	8
8	9	2	6	1	3	4	5	7
7	5	1	2	4	9	8	6	3
3	4	6	5	7	8	1	2	9
1	8	5	4	6	7	9	3	2
9	7	3	1	8	2	6	4	5
2	6	4	3	9	5	7	8	1

Sudoku Solution 2

6	8	1	3	2	5	4	7	9
5	9	4	8	7	1	3	2	6
2	3	7	9	6	4	1	8	5
4	6	3	2	9	7	8	5	1
9	2	5	1	8	6	7	3	4
1	7	8	4	5	3	9	6	2
8	5	6	7	4	9	2	1	3
7	1	9	6	3	2	5	4	8
3	4	2	5	1	8	6	9	7

Sudoku Solution 3

7	5	1	6	2	9	3	4	8
2	6	9	3	4	8	1	5	7
4	3	8	1	7	5	2	9	6
3	9	2	4	6	7	8	1	5
1	8	6	9	5	3	7	2	4
5	7	4	8	1	2	6	3	9
8	1	5	7	3	4	9	6	2
6	2	7	5	9	1	4	8	3
9	4	3	2	8	6	5	7	1

5

Sudoku Solution 4

3	2	7	9	1	8	4	5	6
1	9	5	6	4	2	7	8	3
8	6	4	7	5	3	9	2	1
9	7	6	5	8	4	1	3	2
4	1	8	3	2	6	5	9	7
5	3	2	1	7	9	8	6	4
6	4	3	8	9	7	2	1	5
7	8	1	2	3	5	6	4	9
2	5	9	4	6	1	3	7	8

6

7

CROCHET: SLIP STITCH, FRONT POST, MAGIC RING

WOODWORKING: BEVEL, BAR CLAMP

POTTERY: BANDING WHEEL, KILN, CERAMIC GLAZE

8

1. a) 1963

2. b) All in the Family

3. d) Sean Connery

4. d) Tennis

5. c) 1989

6. a) Magnavox Odyssey

7. c) George Harrison

8. b) Margaret Thatcher

9. a) Volkswagen Beetle

10. b) Gabriel García Márquez

9

A) XL (40)

B) XXVII (27)

C) XXXVI (36)

D) XVIII (18)

E) L (50)

F) LXXIV (74)

10

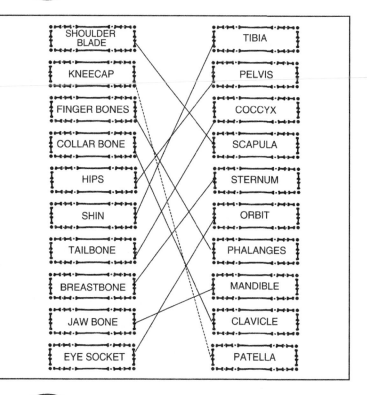

11

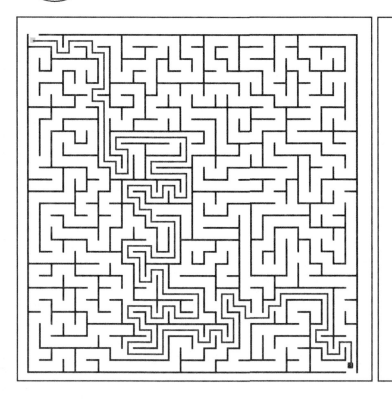

12

Sudoku Solution 5

5	8	7	6	3	4	2	1	9
2	3	6	1	9	7	5	4	8
1	4	9	8	2	5	6	3	7
9	7	1	4	6	3	8	5	2
3	6	4	5	8	2	9	7	1
8	2	5	7	1	9	3	6	4
4	5	2	9	7	6	1	8	3
7	9	8	3	5	1	4	2	6
6	1	3	2	4	8	7	9	5

12

Sudoku Solution 6

6	1	8	4	2	5	7	9	3
9	4	3	6	7	1	8	5	2
2	5	7	8	9	3	4	6	1
3	8	1	5	6	2	9	4	7
7	6	5	9	1	4	2	3	8
4	9	2	7	3	8	6	1	5
1	7	6	3	8	9	5	2	4
5	3	9	2	4	7	1	8	6
8	2	4	1	5	6	3	7	9

Sudoku Solution 7

7	3	4	2	6	8	1	5	9
2	5	8	9	3	1	6	4	7
6	9	1	5	4	7	2	8	3
4	7	9	3	2	5	8	6	1
8	6	5	4	1	9	7	3	2
1	2	3	8	7	6	5	9	4
9	1	6	7	8	3	4	2	5
5	4	7	6	9	2	3	1	8
3	8	2	1	5	4	9	7	6

13

Sudoku Solution 8

5	7	8	1	2	3	9	4	6
6	1	4	9	8	5	3	7	2
9	3	2	4	7	6	5	1	8
3	9	1	2	5	7	8	6	4
7	8	5	6	1	4	2	3	9
2	4	6	8	3	9	7	5	1
4	2	7	3	9	1	6	8	5
1	5	9	7	6	8	4	2	3
8	6	3	5	4	2	1	9	7

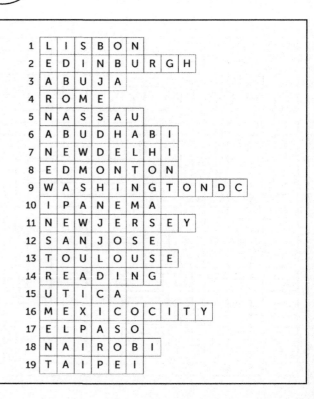

1. LISBON
2. EDINBURGH
3. ABUJA
4. ROME
5. NASSAU
6. ABUDHABI
7. NEWDELHI
8. EDMONTON
9. WASHINGTONDC
10. IPANEMA
11. NEWJERSEY
12. SANJOSE
13. TOULOUSE
14. READING
15. UTICA
16. MEXICOCITY
17. ELPASO
18. NAIROBI
19. TAIPEI

1. Answer: $180,000

Explanation: Multiply the monthly pension amount by 12 months: 2,500 × 12 = 30,000. Then multiply by 6 years: 30,000 x 6 = $180,000

2. Answer: $32,071.74

Explanation: You can use the formula for compound interest: $A = P \times (1+r)n$ where A is the amount accumulated after n years, including interest; P is the principal amount ($10,000); r is the annual interest rate, (6% or 0.06), and n is the number of years (20).
So, A=10,000 x (1 + 0.06)20 = 32,071.74.

3. Answer: $192,000

Explanation: Multiply the monthly annuity payment by the number of months (20 years × 12 months/ year = 240 months): 800 x 240 = 192,000.

4. Answer: $1,800

Explanation: 60,000 x 0.06 = 3600. The employer will match 50% of this amount, which is 3600 x 0.5 = 1800.

14

5. Answer: $579.64

Explanation: You can use the formula for compound interest: A = P × (1+r)n, where A is the amount after n years, P = 500, r = 3% or 0.03, and n = 5.
So, A = 500 x (1 + 0.03)5

15

ASTRONAUT

SUPERNOVA

SATELLITE

ANDROMEDA

ASTEROIDS

TELESCOPE

16

A) PANAMA

B) AUSTRALIA

C) BRAZIL

D) FRANCE

E) ITALY

17

```
I D P Z F R U I T I F X G H L N A R A I
H Y T P L X S U N L I G H T G M U E G X
F G Z M O Z G E P S B P X E R K H K Q I
F D B J W L O T E V E R G R E E N U H R
O A A C E W L D R D A V E G E T A B L E
E S X R R H U I E B L F D K N H B T L K
T H O W S E Y Z N N C I O H H R D W J M
L E R I D E V G N A H L N F O R K F R Z
M A X A L L U T I P T A M G U T P P P D
V R P W A B H R A Q D I I W S A L S O N
Y S N W Y A J O L B A I O O E I P N O W
V M B D L R Y W S W R V P N L E K X N L
L V A D G R F E D E O M L G C W D S T M
P L N N Z O M L G H O P R U N E R S Z P
G A E O U W R K E C T P H E P K B K O Y
T W A T E R I N G C A N D E E H L Z C H
Z I I W Y S E E D S D Q O W F U Y R O T
```

18

HORROR: THE BIRDS, THE OMEN, SUSPIRIA

ROMANCE: MOONSTRUCK, NOTTING HILL, MYSTIC PIZZA

FANTASY: TIME BANDITS, THE WIZ

19

BUENOS AIRES

LOS ANGELES

RIO DE JANIERO

HAVANA

NEW ORLEANS

VANCOUVER

BARRANQUILLA

MONTREAL

20

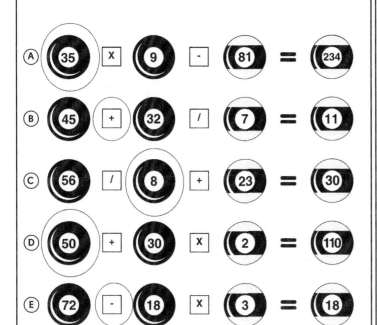

21

A) PANAMA

B) BARBADOS

C) KENYA

D) SOUTH AFRICA

E) SOUTH KOREA

F) PAKISTAN

G) ARGENTINA

H) CAMBODIA

I) PORTUGAL

J) CHILE

22

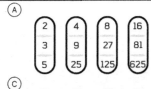

Ⓑ
2 3 4 | 5 8 11 | 10 15 20 | 17 24 31

Ⓒ
1 2 3 | 3 6 9 | 7 12 21 | 13 20 35

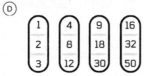

A) First Row: Each number is a power of 2.
Second Row: Each number is a power of 3.
Third Row: Each number is a power of 5.
B) Row 1: Start from 2, increment by 3, 5, and 7.
Row 2: Start from 3, increment by 5, 7, and 9.
Row 3: Start from 4, increment by 7, 9, and 11.

C) Column 1: Start from 1, increment by 2, 3, and 4.
Column 2: Start from 3, increment by 4, 6, and 8.
Column 3: Start from 7, increment by 6, 12, and 14.
Column 4: Start from 13, increment by 7, 8, and 16.
D) Each number is calculated by multiplying the row number with the square of the column number.

Sudoku Solution 9

2	3	7	4	1	9	5	8	6
6	8	1	3	5	2	7	9	4
5	4	9	7	6	8	1	2	3
7	5	2	6	8	4	9	3	1
8	9	6	1	7	3	2	4	5
3	1	4	2	9	5	8	6	7
9	6	5	8	3	1	4	7	2
1	2	3	9	4	7	6	5	8
4	7	8	5	2	6	3	1	9

Sudoku Solution 10

5	4	9	1	3	6	8	2	7
8	1	6	2	7	4	3	5	9
3	2	7	9	8	5	1	6	4
7	3	1	4	2	9	5	8	6
2	9	5	7	6	8	4	1	3
4	6	8	5	1	3	9	7	2
9	8	2	6	4	1	7	3	5
1	7	4	3	5	2	6	9	8
6	5	3	8	9	7	2	4	1

Sudoku Solution 11

1	7	2	8	3	6	4	9	5
4	9	8	1	2	5	6	7	3
3	6	5	4	7	9	8	2	1
2	5	9	3	6	1	7	4	8
8	1	6	7	5	4	2	3	9
7	3	4	2	9	8	5	1	6
9	8	7	6	1	2	3	5	4
5	4	3	9	8	7	1	6	2
6	2	1	5	4	3	9	8	7

Sudoku Solution 12

3	4	6	2	7	9	5	1	8
2	1	9	5	6	8	3	7	4
7	8	5	1	3	4	6	9	2
5	7	3	8	2	1	9	4	6
1	2	8	9	4	6	7	5	3
6	9	4	3	5	7	8	2	1
8	5	2	7	1	3	4	6	9
9	6	7	4	8	2	1	3	5
4	3	1	6	9	5	2	8	7

1. a) Fonzie

2. c) Brady

3. d) Sherman Hemsley

4. c) Cheers

5. a) Mr. Roper

6. c) Robin Williams

7. c) The Andy Griffith Show

8. a) Gary Coleman

9. d) Marcia

10.b) Jean Stapleton

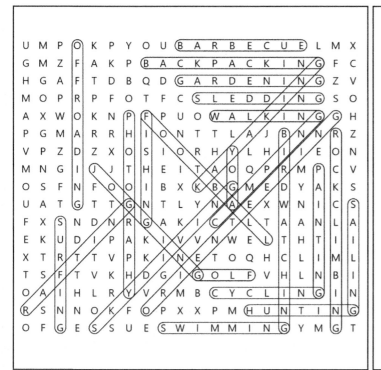

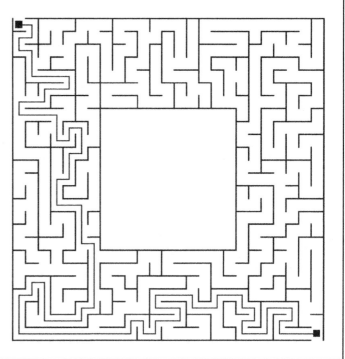

25

27

A) INTERCEPTION

B) RED ZONE

C) FAIR CATCH

28

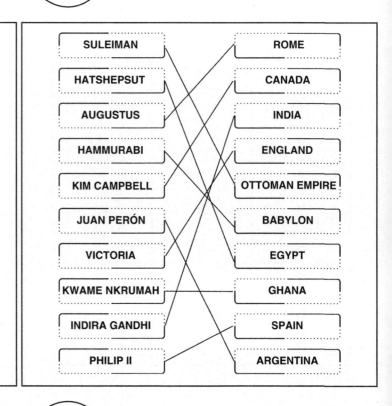

SULEIMAN	ROME
HATSHEPSUT	CANADA
AUGUSTUS	INDIA
HAMMURABI	ENGLAND
KIM CAMPBELL	OTTOMAN EMPIRE
JUAN PERÓN	BABYLON
VICTORIA	EGYPT
KWAME NKRUMAH	GHANA
INDIRA GANDHI	SPAIN
PHILIP II	ARGENTINA

29

A) FALL OF BERLIN WALL

B) GREAT DEPRESSION

C) SPACE RACE

D) FORMATION OF THE EU

30

A) -

B) 7

C) 96

D) 10

E) 4

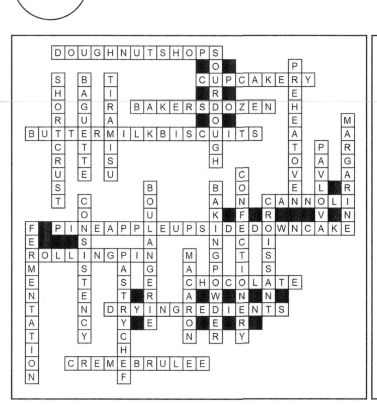

1. Answer = $24,466.51

Explanation: You can use the formula for compound interest:
$A = P \times (1+r)n$ to solve.

2. Answer = $576,000

Explanation: Multiply the monthly pension amount by the number of months in 15 years.

3. Answer: $35,000

Explanation: Multiply the annual vacation budget by the number of years.

32

4. Answer: $9,000

Explanation: Multiply the monthly expense by the number of months in 5 years.

5. Answer: $300,000

Explanation: Multiply the annual benefit by the number of years.

33

A) LXXIX (79)

B) LV (55)

C) LIV (54)

D) XXX (30)

E) XXXVII (37)

F) XLV (45)

34

NORTH AMERICA: MOUNT WHITNEY, DENALI, MOUNT LOGAN

EUROPE: MONT BLANC, MATTERHORN, BEN NEVIS

AFRICA: MOUNT STANLEY, KILIMANJARO

35

A) CHEESES

B) EMERGENCY SERVICES

C) DESERT

D) CITRUS FRUITS

E) BREADS

36

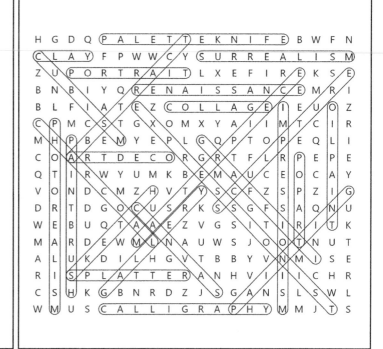

37

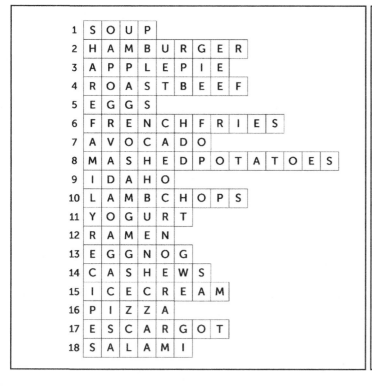

1. SOUP
2. HAMBURGER
3. APPLEPIE
4. ROASTBEEF
5. EGGS
6. FRENCHFRIES
7. AVOCADO
8. MASHEDPOTATOES
9. IDAHO
10. LAMBCHOPS
11. YOGURT
12. RAMEN
13. EGGNOG
14. CASHEWS
15. ICECREAM
16. PIZZA
17. ESCARGOT
18. SALAMI

38

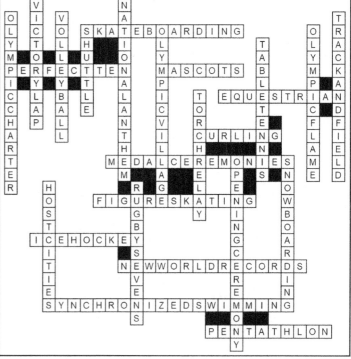

39

CROSSHATCH

EXHIBITION

ILLUSTRATE

PAINTBRUSH

MASTERPIECE

SCULPTURES

40

A) XLI (41)

B) XLVIII (48)

C) XXII (22)

D) XLV (45)

E) LXXXI (81)

F) XXXVII (37)

41

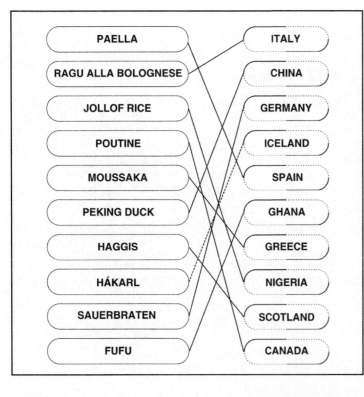

PAELLA	ITALY
RAGU ALLA BOLOGNESE	CHINA
JOLLOF RICE	GERMANY
POUTINE	ICELAND
MOUSSAKA	SPAIN
PEKING DUCK	GHANA
HAGGIS	GREECE
HÁKARL	NIGERIA
SAUERBRATEN	SCOTLAND
FUFU	CANADA

42

```
F A W L T Y T O W E R S F R S P F Q B G
G A M G G M A U D E B L A C K A D D E R
J T M X A I X M R N I G H T C O U R T C
N H E A N U I E R W T P D K M X D A H H
H E A N L D F U L L H O U S E Q O W R S
C F N F I Y S G S F E K S E Z B P U E T
X A F H N O M A N N G O M T E S G M E H
Z C O E T U G A P H O B P V O I D S E
I T R D O H R M T T Z L W O T V T K H C
E S D D E R L Q R G T D L J H D P K A O
I O A D F A F C H E E R S O A B B P M
S N N C A N D W C H N R O O B X L P A
J L D O M G I T A G G S O K G U Y Y N
R I S U I L Q R B I O W M V V E D A Y
E F O P L A A D J V R C L Z O Y J A
G E N L Y G L Z X A L L O A L L O Y K
M T H E J E F F E R S O N S F X D S E
```

43

CRAYFISH

FLY FISHING

ANGLING

SALMON

FRESHWATER

CRUSTACEAN

BOBBER

SINKER

44

A) ANGLES

B) FISHING STYLES

C) TYPES OF WINE

D) SOCIAL MEDIA SITE FOUNDERS

E) BRITISH AUTHORS

45

A) XL (40)

B) XVIII (18)

C) XXX (30)

D) LXXV (75)

E) LV (55)

F) XXIV (24)

46

1. b) Gardening

2. c) Crochet

3. d) Reading

4. b) Woodworking

5. d) Fishing

6. a) Flower arranging

7. a) Pottery

8. c) Stamp collecting

9. c) Sewing

10.c) Scrapbooking

A) LAUNCH OF SPUTNIK

B) INVENTION OF THE INTERNET

C) CHERNOBYL DISASTER

A) MAYA ANGELOU

B) ROBERT FROST

C) RUMI

1. Answer = $44,081.63

Explanation: You can use the formula for compound interest: $A = P \times (1+r)n$ to solve.

2. Answer: 314 square ft.

Explanation: Calculate the area of each section and add them together: 15 x 10 = 150, 12 x 9 = 108, 8 x 7 = 56.
Total area = 150 + 108 + 56 = 314.

3. Answer: 96 hours

Explanation: Number of rounds per week: 3, Hours per round: 4, Weeks: 8. Total hours: 3 × 4 × 8 = 96 hours.

4. Answer: 17.5 cups

Explanation: Cups of flour per batch: 2.5, Number of batches: 7. Total cups of flour: 2.5 × 7 = 17.5 cups.

50

5. Answer: 20 hours
Explanation: Games per week: 2, Hours per game: 2.5, Weeks in a month: 4.
Total hours: 2 × 2.5 × 4 = 20 hours.

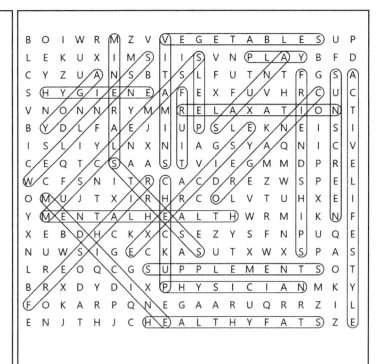

51

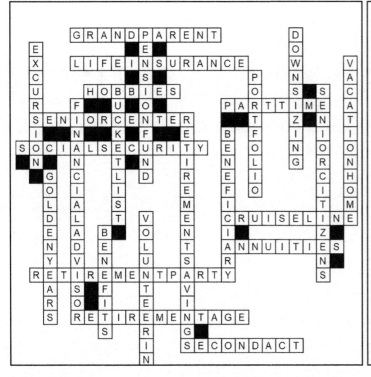

52

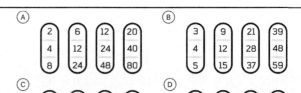

A) Row 1: Start with 2, adding 4, 6, and 8.
Row 2: Start with 4, adding 8, 12, and 16.
Row 3: Start with 8, adding 16, 24, and 32.
B) Row 1: Start from 3, increment by 6, 12, and 18.
Row 2: Start from 4, increment by 8, 16, and 20.

Row 3: Start from 5, increment by 10, 22, and 22.
C) Row 1: 1+4, 1+8, 1+16, 1+24
Row 2: 3+6, 3+12, 3+18, 3+24
Row3: 5+10, 5+20, 5+28, 5+30
D) Row 1 : Powers of 2
Row 2: Powers of 3
Row 3: Powers of 4

53

A) 3

B) 45

C) -

D) 15

E) +

54

A) JAPAN

B) MEXICO

C) ARGENTINA

D) IRELAND

E) SOUTH AFRICA

55

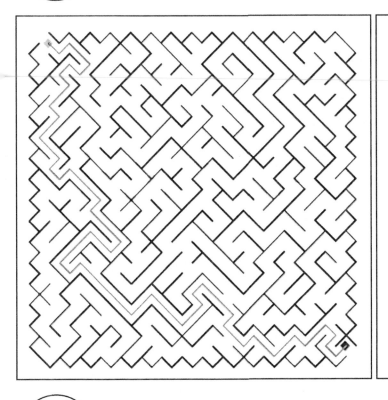

56

A) LVI (56)

B) XCVIII (98)

C) XCII (92)

D) CVII (107)

E) LXXIX (79)

F) LIV (54)

57

Sudoku Solution 13

6	2	1	8	5	9	7	4	3
3	8	9	4	7	2	5	6	1
7	4	5	1	6	3	9	2	8
8	9	6	2	1	7	4	3	5
4	7	2	5	3	6	8	1	9
1	5	3	9	4	8	6	7	2
5	3	7	6	8	1	2	9	4
9	6	8	3	2	4	1	5	7
2	1	4	7	9	5	3	8	6

Sudoku Solution 14

4	8	3	6	2	7	9	1	5
7	6	2	5	9	1	3	4	8
5	9	1	4	8	3	7	6	2
8	2	4	9	3	6	1	5	7
9	1	7	8	4	5	6	2	3
6	3	5	7	1	2	4	8	9
3	4	9	2	6	8	5	7	1
1	5	8	3	7	4	2	9	6
2	7	6	1	5	9	8	3	4

57

Sudoku Solution 15

4	7	2	1	9	6	8	5	3
5	8	9	3	4	2	1	6	7
6	1	3	7	8	5	4	2	9
2	3	6	9	1	4	7	8	5
7	5	1	8	2	3	9	4	6
9	4	8	5	6	7	3	1	2
3	9	4	6	5	1	2	7	8
1	6	7	2	3	8	5	9	4
8	2	5	4	7	9	6	3	1

Sudoku Solution 16

4	5	9	2	3	8	6	1	7
1	8	6	4	5	7	3	9	2
7	2	3	1	9	6	4	8	5
6	7	1	9	8	4	2	5	3
5	9	2	3	7	1	8	6	4
3	4	8	5	6	2	1	7	9
8	1	4	7	2	5	9	3	6
2	3	7	6	1	9	5	4	8
9	6	5	8	4	3	7	2	1

58

SLIP STITCH

FAIR ISLE

CABLE

LEADING LEG

BIND OFF

CAST ON

NEEDLES

BACKSTITCH

59

CHECKERS

SCRABBLE

MONOPOLY

GUESS WHO

SEQUENCE

CONNECT 4

60

A) LAIKA

B) HARAMBE

C) SECRETARIAT

61

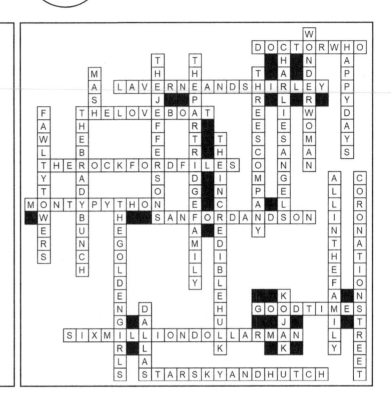

62

1. Answer: 60 fish

Explanation: Fish per hour: 5, Hours per day: 6, Days: 2. Total fish: 5 × 6 × 2 = 60 fish.

2. Answer: 24 days

Explanation: Pages per day: 50, Pages per book: 300. Days per book: 300 / 50 = 6 days. For 4 books: 6 × 4 = 24 days.

62

3. Answer: 4 days

Explanation: Total miles: 1,200, Miles per hour: 60, Hours per day: 5. Miles per day: 60 × 5 = 300 miles. Days: 1,200 / 300 = 4 days.

4. Answer: 9 yards

Explanation: Yards of yarn per foot: 1.5, Length of scarf: 6 feet. Total yards of yarn: 1.5 × 6 = 9 yards.

5. Answer: 6 hours

Explanation: Minutes per game: 90, Games: 4. Total minutes: 90 × 4 = 360 minutes. Convert to hours: 360 / 60 = 6 hours.

63

```
I F Q E G E S B P S T R U M P K I Z F Z
P N J V L E S S O N S R H E E F F B U G
V T R E A Z W D Z Z A H F T R L I R H K
D T R R B N W D C W X Y T R J R O C K V
G U I T A R K D C O O T D O W X T D K K
B C X E P Q X Y L O P H O N E I N R Y E
A L F M T X F L B R H M K O P D M U O K
B A G P I P E S S A O A P M I T Z M P O
I S G O S C A L E P N A R E A T V X C V
K S H Z C V B B N I E D A M N W Y J Y O
R I K S H E E T M U S I C G O R O T E Z
E C K I M P R O V I S A T I O N U M Z P
I A N C O M P O S I T I O N L Y A E I
R U C U K K A Q N I E L C D R F J J S X
P N D J I R F T R U M P E T W E Q G T A
A W R Q R W T H A F B A K Z S H D G F P
D X Y B Z I K P O F K K T I D O L B O N
```

64

PERSIA: FARSI , KURDISH, TAJIK

JAPAN: OKINAWAN, AMAMI

SPAIN: CASTILIAN, CATALAN, GALICIAN

65

A) DIWALI

B) BEACHES

C) PONY BREEDS

D) MOLLUSCS

E) FRUITS

66

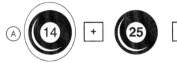 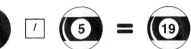
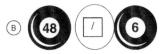 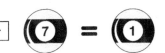
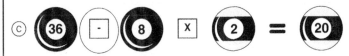
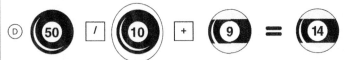
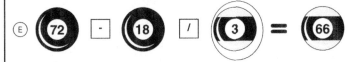

A) 14 + 25 / 5 = 19

B) 48 / 6 - 7 = 1

C) 36 - 8 X 2 = 20

D) 50 / 10 + 9 = 14

E) 72 - 18 / 3 = 66

67

A) MALALA YOUSAFZAI

B) W.E.B. DU BOIS

C) JANE FONDA

68

A) ISLANDS OF THE HEBRIDES

B) CHEWING GUM BRANDS

C) THE WIZARD OF OZ

D) TYPES OF JAZZ

E) VOCAL SOUNDS

69

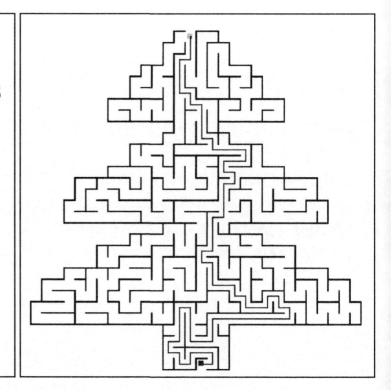

70

```
S O J P O W E R S U I T M D Z C W X F A
S C E W S K I N N Y J E A N S A F L I V
G P L E G H S P A N D E X M T T N P I I
V N L P V P O N C H O S I B I E Y E A A
U W Y A I X S U Q Y R Z S A B Y H A T T
B B S T T U H M L E F M K A G I E A S O
R A A C I F D O F D O J I K G W A N U R
Y L N H R B O A T T E M R Y L I A T N S
B L D W E S O R T P Q R T J N I B L U U
M E A O N L A O M R A U P E I S A L O N
W T L R C K B M F S A N T A T S E L V G
H F S K Q L Z F B E H C T N D E N O I L
W L E J L Q T Y P D Q O K S D S S U V A
X A F E D O R A W U V X E S Q D H S E S
R T B A L E G W A R M E R S U K I E S S
E S Q N D D Y K Z M I N I S K I R T S E
Z X O S L E A T H E R J A C K E T V T S
```

71

1. b) Minecraft

2. a) Frozen

3. a) Hogwarts

4. a) Ryder

5. a) Transformers

6. c) TikTok

7. d) Pokémon World

8. b) Harry Potter

9. a) Pig

10. a) Floss

Sudoku Solution 17

7	1	9	4	6	2	3	5	8
3	8	2	1	5	9	7	6	4
4	5	6	3	8	7	2	9	1
8	6	3	2	9	5	4	1	7
2	9	5	7	4	1	8	3	6
1	4	7	6	3	8	9	2	5
6	7	8	9	1	3	5	4	2
9	2	1	5	7	4	6	8	3
5	3	4	8	2	6	1	7	9

Sudoku Solution 18

6	8	7	9	2	4	1	5	3
5	4	1	7	8	3	2	9	6
3	2	9	1	6	5	4	8	7
1	7	2	5	4	6	9	3	8
4	6	5	3	9	8	7	2	1
8	9	3	2	7	1	6	4	5
2	3	6	8	1	9	5	7	4
7	5	4	6	3	2	8	1	9
9	1	8	4	5	7	3	6	2

Sudoku Solution 19

9	8	3	7	4	6	5	1	2
7	5	2	8	9	1	4	3	6
1	4	6	3	5	2	7	8	9
6	1	5	2	8	9	3	7	4
2	3	4	6	1	7	9	5	8
8	9	7	5	3	4	2	6	1
5	7	9	1	2	8	6	4	3
4	6	1	9	7	3	8	2	5
3	2	8	4	6	5	1	9	7

Sudoku Solution 20

7	5	1	6	9	2	8	4	3
3	6	4	1	7	8	2	9	5
2	8	9	5	3	4	1	6	7
8	4	6	2	5	3	9	7	1
9	2	7	8	1	6	3	5	4
1	3	5	7	4	9	6	2	8
6	1	3	4	2	5	7	8	9
4	9	8	3	6	7	5	1	2
5	7	2	9	8	1	4	3	6

BIRDIE

CADDIE

GREENS

GOLFER

DRIVER

PUTTER

MALLET

TEE BOX

MARKER

#										
1	B	E	E	S						
2	U	N	D	E	R					
3	I	N	S	U	R	A	N	C	E	
4	L	I	O	N						
5	D	R	I	V	E					
6	I	V	O	R	Y					
7	N	O	T	H	I	N	G			
8	G	U	M	B	Y					
9	A	N	T							
10	T	O	M	A	T	O				
11	R	A	B	I	D					
12	E	C	O	L	O	G	Y			
13	E	L	E	V	A	T	I	O	N	
14	H	O	M	E	R					
15	O	C	T	O	P	U	S			
16	U	K	U	L	E	L	E			
17	S	P	I	D	E	R	M	A	N	
18	E	V	E	R	E	S	T			

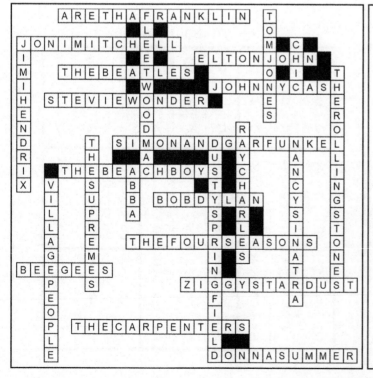

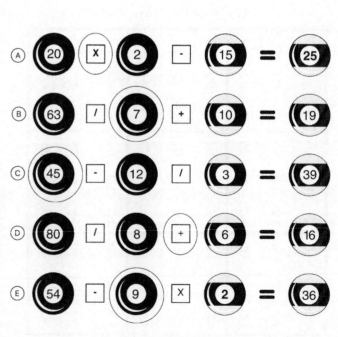

A) 20 X 2 - 15 = 25

B) 63 / 7 + 10 = 19

C) 45 - 12 / 3 = 39

D) 80 / 8 + 6 = 16

E) 54 - 9 X 2 = 36

1. Answer: $40

Explanation: Sets of photographs: 5, Cost per set: $8. Total cost: 5 × 8 = $40.

2. Answer: 90 hours

Explanation: Hours per day: 3, Days per week: 5. Weekly hours: 3 × 5 = 15. Total weeks: 6. Total hours: 15 × 6 = 90 hours.

3. Answer: 144 bird species

Explanation: Bird species per outing: 12, Outings per month: 4. Monthly total: 12 × 4 = 48. Total months: 3. Total species: 48 × 3 = 144.

4. Answer: 30 cups of sugar

Explanation: Cups of sugar per batch: 0.75, Batches per week: 10. Weekly total: 0.75 × 10 = 7.5. Total weeks: 4. Total sugar: 7.5 × 4 = 30 cups.

77

5. Answer: 24 hours

Explanation: Hours per day: 2, Days per week: 3 (Monday, Wednesday, Friday). Weekly total: 2 × 3 = 6. Total weeks: 4. Total hours: 6 × 4 = 24 hours.

78

A) BRANDENBURG GATE

B) STONEHENGE

C) SISTINE CHAPEL

79

OPENING OF DISNEY WORLD	2004
MOON LANDING	1969
LAUNCH OF FACEBOOK	2010
DEATH OF PRINCESS DIANA	1985
CHALLENGER DISASTER	1997
THATCHER BECOMES U.K PM	1971
FALL OF THE BERLIN WALL	1986
LAUNCH OF PLAYSTATION 1	1979
LIVE AID CONCERT	1989
LAUNCH OF THE IPAD	1994

80

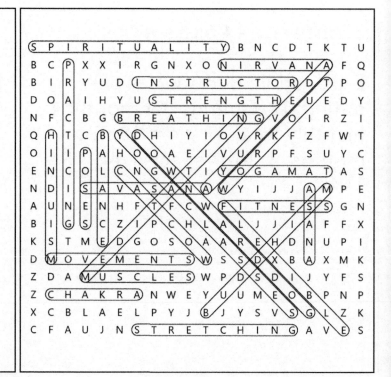

A) XXX (30)

B) XVIII (18)

C) XX (20)

D) LX (60)

E) XXI (21)

F) XL (40)

A) GREEK GODS

B) FICTIONAL DETECTIVES

C) DANCE MOVES

D) AMERICAN INDUSTRIES

E) FAMOUS LEES

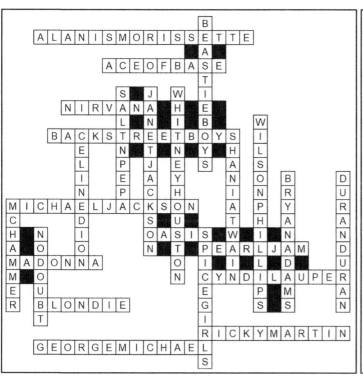

(A) 1 4 9 16 / 2 8 18 32 / 3 12 27 48

(B) 2 5 8 11 / 4 8 12 16 / 6 12 18 24

(C) 1 3 5 7 / 2 6 10 14 / 4 12 20 28

(D) 1 3 7 13 / 2 6 12 20 / 5 15 29 45

A) Each number is the product of the row number and the square of the column number.

B) Each number is the sum of the row number and an increasing sequence based on the column.

C) Row 1: Start from 1, increase by 2 each time.
Row 2: Start from 2, increase by 4 each time.

Row 3: Start from 4, increase by 8 each time.
D) Row 1: Starts at 1, with differences increasing by 2 (2, 4, 6).
Row 2: Starts at 2, with differences increasing by 4 (4, 6, 8).
Row 3: Starts at 5, with differences increasing by 10 (10, 14, 16).

85

MEDITATION

SACRED

DIVINE

SUPERNATURAL

WORSHIP

ASTROLOGY

SCRIPTURE

HEAVEN

86

1. b) Platform shoes

2. a) Denim

3. a) Bell-bottoms

4. b) Shag

5. d) Newsboy cap

6. a) Maxi dress

7. a) Bandana

8. d) Denim jacket

9. c) Clogs

10. c) Wide collar

87

BRAZIL: BELO HORIZONTE, SALVADOR

GERMANY: DRESDEN, COLOGNE, FRANKFURT

FRANCE: GRENOBLE, DIJON, STRASBOURG

88

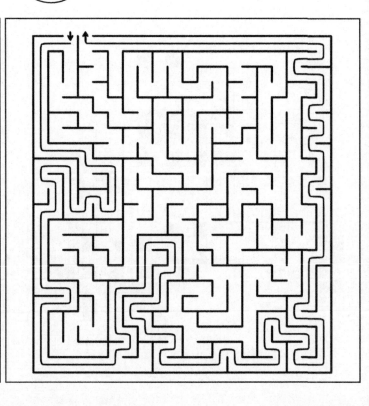

89

```
M M G S O D C M F M Y (A L E X A N D E R)
R K S E G H B I Z (C D R) Z D Y G S C T T
Z J A D N J V Z D L L D H Z L Q O K F L
Q A S C E G K (R A M S E S) G B X A M D X
V D C A H G H J A W O R O F P S E L O L
(C Y R U S) U A I F J M N V P E L O W O L
O B U A I B R U S K R L T I A O M A O
X O O I T O W C L K E S Z V R T E T N
M F G L T S Z H H L H N H X S C R N E A
E E L C I B Z U P I E A N I O D K A V
U J I F N V M V D M L I N E N R E P J
L V N J G A Q R A D L P O D Z L O L Q
Z J C G B I D R M N H W X B N Y O L T H
S P O S U I L U A D B M N A Q B O E J N
X H L L L I O H (J E F F E R S O N) O P L
Z L N J L U G K I L C I O (M E L O N I) T
P J R W R I E (T H A T C H E R) W O B C Y
```

90

Sudoku Solution 21

8	2	4	6	5	1	9	7	3
3	9	6	7	4	8	1	5	2
5	7	1	2	3	9	4	6	8
9	6	5	3	7	4	8	2	1
4	8	3	1	2	5	7	9	6
7	1	2	9	8	6	3	4	5
1	4	8	5	9	2	6	3	7
2	3	9	8	6	7	5	1	4
6	5	7	4	1	3	2	8	9

Sudoku Solution 22

2	1	3	8	9	5	7	4	6
9	6	5	2	4	7	3	1	8
7	8	4	1	3	6	2	9	5
5	7	1	4	6	3	8	2	9
3	4	8	7	2	9	6	5	1
6	2	9	5	8	1	4	7	3
1	9	6	3	7	2	5	8	4
8	5	7	6	1	4	9	3	2
4	3	2	9	5	8	1	6	7

Sudoku Solution 23

5	4	3	2	9	1	7	6	8
8	7	6	3	4	5	1	2	9
1	9	2	8	6	7	5	3	4
3	5	9	6	7	2	4	8	1
6	1	7	5	8	4	3	9	2
2	8	4	9	1	3	6	7	5
4	6	1	7	2	8	9	5	3
9	3	8	1	5	6	2	4	7
7	2	5	4	3	9	8	1	6

90

Sudoku Solution 24

9	2	1	8	6	4	5	7	3
4	8	7	9	5	3	2	6	1
5	3	6	7	2	1	8	4	9
6	9	4	5	3	8	7	1	2
3	1	8	2	4	7	6	9	5
7	5	2	1	9	6	3	8	4
2	4	9	6	7	5	1	3	8
1	7	3	4	8	2	9	5	6
8	6	5	3	1	9	4	2	7

91

FORD: MUSTANG, RANGER, THUNDERBIRD

CHEVROLET: CORVETTE, SILVERADO

VOLKSWAGEN: TRANSPORTER, BEETLE, GOLF

92

1. LLAMA
2. ELEPHANT
3. APPLE
4. RAPTORS
5. NATALIE
6. IGUANA
7. NEWTON
8. GROVER
9. AGAVE
10. NOTION
11. ELVIS
12. WEST INDIES
13. ILLEGAL
14. NEVERLAND
15. SELDOM
16. TARANTINO
17. RICKY
18. UFC
19. MANGO
20. ELEMENT
21. NEWBIE
22. TALENT

93

A) MEDICAL SCIENTISTS

B) DESCRIPTIONS OF MEN

C) FROG SPECIES

D) FAMOUS PAINTINGS

E) HIKING TRAILS IN THE U.S.A

94

AFRICA: ANCIENT EGYPT, AKSUM, KUSH

THE AMERICAS: AZTEC, MAYA, OLMEC

ASIA: HARAPPA, QIN DYNASTY

95

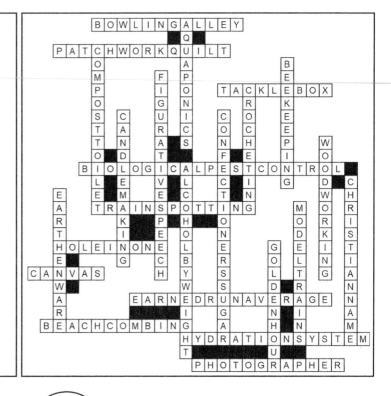

96

CRUISE

STREEP

WEAVER

WALKEN

PACINO

SNIPES

SEAGAL

NORRIS

CURTIS

97

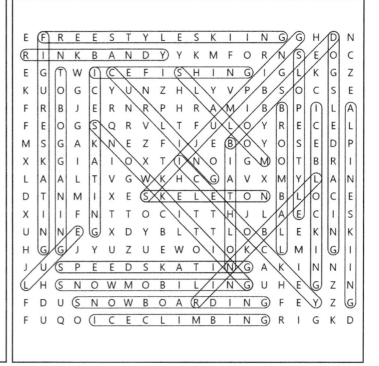

98

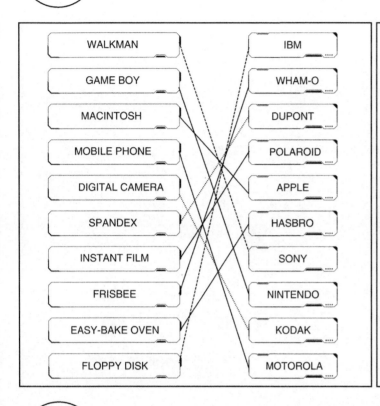

WALKMAN	IBM
GAME BOY	WHAM-O
MACINTOSH	DUPONT
MOBILE PHONE	POLAROID
DIGITAL CAMERA	APPLE
SPANDEX	HASBRO
INSTANT FILM	SONY
FRISBEE	NINTENDO
EASY-BAKE OVEN	KODAK
FLOPPY DISK	MOTOROLA

99

A) -

B) 25

C) 5

D) 3

E) 4

100

INVESTMENT

PENSION

INSURANCE

TRAVEL

ASSETS

FAMILY

EXPAT

CRUISE

101

A) FAMOUS SCULPTURES

B) FAMOUS DOGS

C) KEANU REEVES MOVIES

D) SPORTS PLAYED WITH A NET

E) FAMOUS PHILOSOPHERS

Printed in Great Britain
by Amazon

56072679R00097